Getting Great Spa

On the Road to Wellness

Spa Well
Live long
Kathryn Stacee

Stolle Service Ltd.,
1360 Rockland Avenue, Victoria, B.C., Canada
250-370-2727 or online at info@stolle.com

Cover design and layout: Rick Stolle

www.stolle.com

ISBN 978-0-9878457-0-2
ISBN 978-0-9878457-1-9 (e-book)

Printed in the United States of America

10 9 8 7 6 5 4 3 2

For my wonderful husband Rick

Table of Contents

Foreword by Susie Ellis

Everyone notices when Kathryn Stolle walks into a room. She is tall, fit, beautiful, has the most wonderful skin, and wow – that hair! Kathryn juggles a busy life with her husband of over forty years, family and a full-time career – all the while exuding confidence, wisdom, and immeasurable happiness. Her inner calm and outer joy is the radiant result of living a healthy, spa-inspired lifestyle.

Last summer, Kathryn shared with me the preliminary manuscript for this book, *Getting Great Spa*. When I first picked it up, I expected to find it full of information for first-time spa-goers, or people who simply want to get more out of their spa experiences. It does all that for sure. But I was also pleasantly surprised that it resonates with more seasoned spa-goers and spa professionals like me.

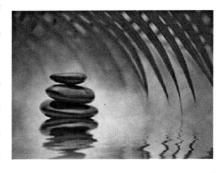

Kathryn and I have known each other for decades and laughingly agree that, when it comes to the modern spa industry, we have pretty much been there from the get-go. Being a matchmaker of sorts for people and spas most of my life, I can honestly say that finding the right spa, wellness experience or regime can be as important as finding the right life partner. It can change everything! After decades of seeing people emerge from spas looking fantastic and feeling their best, I've come to the conclusion that spas are the best places to make lasting lifestyle changes – and they also happen to be extremely comfortable, nurturing and, in many cases, fun.

The spa industry itself has gone through some transformation in the last 30 years. Today, there are over 80,000 spas globally, and, in the U.S. alone, there are now more spas than there are Starbucks in the world! Spa going, once narrowly associated with wealthy women, pampering and luxury, has been transformed into an utterly mainstream activity, attracting people of all genders, ages, classes, nations and races. Furthermore, spas have vastly expanded their offerings beyond massage and facials, to embrace so many new wellness and beauty offerings: from fitness, yoga and alternative medicine – to medically supervised procedures.

So many spas…so many choices…that's why the pages of this book are the perfect guide in helping you understand and navigate these rich, amazing offerings at the modern spa, identify what spas and experiences are ideal for you and learn how to truly maximize the value of the activities and treatments you embrace. Kathryn has accomplished something that I think hasn't been done before: writing a book that will be enjoyed by, and be of value to, anyone wanting to get an insider's view of the world of spas.

As you turn the pages of this book, moving from chapter to chapter, you will feel Kathryn becoming a close friend, one you can look to for inspiration and advice. Taking this journey will not only be educational but also enjoyable. It is my hope that by the time you finish the last chapter that you will be able to join the group of us who say, with enthusiasm and confidence, "we do know how to get great spa!"

Susie Ellis

Susie Ellis, President of SpaFinder, Inc., the world's largest spa media and marketing company that celebrated its 25th anniversary in 2011, is a highly respected authority and analyst of the global spa, wellness and beauty industries, a member of the Board of Directors of the Global Spa Summit and author of the definitive annual "Spa Trends Forecast."

Chapter 1   What's in a Name?   Defining Spa

I love Spas and everything about them! It doesn't matter whether they're big or small, day or stay, posh or simple – when I find one that's well run and staffed by people who care, something inside of me shouts "Yes!" Sure I can "spa at home," but as far as I'm concerned, it can't compare with the magic and inspiration I find in the spa.

What It Is and What it Does

But what is a spa? Where does a salon end and a day spa begin? Can a hotel with a swimming pool, hot tub and a couple of massage rooms call these amenities a spa? Or when a resort hotel has a full complement of spa facilities

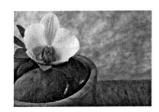

and programs can it refer to itself as a destination spa? To get great spa, you need to know the answers to these and a host of other questions.

In 1997, the Board of Directors of the International Spa Association met in Boston to define the term "Spa." This proved to be no easy task. There were some who maintained that a spa must include water – in some form – in its treatments, while others claimed that water wasn't necessary to provide a healing or nurturing experience. The lively and animated conversation around the table resulted in a stalemate. "Then why," someone suggested, "don't we define what spa does and not what it is?"

In short order, we came up with a definition of the spa experience that is still valid today: "time to relax, reflect, revitalize and rejoice." Since then, ISPA has further defined Spa (though still without mention of water): "Spas are places devoted to enhancing overall wellbeing through a variety of professional services that encourage renewal of mind, body and spirit."

In other words, regardless of whether you decide to stop for a massage at an airport kiosk or book a week at your favourite destination spa with all the bells and whistles, if you can enhance your wellbeing – your body, your mind and your spirit – you reap the benefits a spa provides.

 Body, Mind, Spirit

Defining Body is a fairly straightforward proposition. The treatments that minister to your body, such as a facial, hot stone massage or pedicure, help your body renew itself in some way. You emerge from the treatment with a glowing complexion, relaxed demeanour or fabulous toes, tangible evidence of the "relax" and "revitalize" aspects of Spa.

Mind is also reasonably easy to define. So many things in a well-appointed spa are designed to quiet and calm the mind by appealing to the senses – soothing music and colour schemes, quiet voices, fragrant scents. Calming your mind allows you to be in the moment and receptive to the energy and ministrations of your therapist, thereby achieving the maximum benefit from your treatment. Sure there are some very busy day spas that seem to be cranking out treatments and services without regard to some of these aspects of spa – but once you're in the privacy of one of their treatment rooms you'll probably experience renewal and relaxation in some way.

Spirit is a far, far more difficult concept to pinpoint or define. It is the essence of your being that responds to the healing power of touch and the sharing of energy during the spa experience. It encompasses your values - how you relate to others and how you embrace ideas and experiences that are meaningful or relevant to you. It is not necessarily "spiritual" in a religious sense, although at times it can be, but it does address the need we all have to feel connected, inspired, uplifted and part of the greater whole.

So consider the benefits of a massage: a more vigorous and robust body; a calmer, more serene mind and/or greater ability to cope with stress; and finally a bounce in your step that comes with feeling refreshed and happy. All three components of Spa have been realized and you are the richer for the experience.

What's the Difference?

Spas are easily divided into two categories: "day spa" or "stay spa." The treatments and services in a day spa are generally provided in the course of a single day and the spa does not offer accommodations; while as the name implies, a stay spa features accommodations along with treatments, programs and a variety of activities.

The following classifications will help you better navigate your way through the maze of descriptions and definitions floating around.

Day Spas

Day spas comprise the majority of (four out of five) spas in North America. They can be found in malls, in homes, as freestanding businesses, in airports and in a variety of other locations. Many started as beauty salons and morphed into the day spas of today, adding treatments and services such as pedicures, massages, body treatments, water-based treatments and specialized facials, often adopting more of a wellness focus. Though they might vary in size or treatment menu, most of them incorporate the "body, mind and spirit" philosophy that sets a spa apart from its salon counterpart.

 From the Beginning

In the early 1900's, Elizabeth Arden opened The Red Door Salon on New York's Fifth Avenue – the precursor of today's day spa. As an independent businesswoman, Arden developed products and services to improve a woman's appearance and express her individuality in the early days of women's suffrage.

Her mantra, "To be beautiful and natural is the birthright of every woman," could have been coined today.

With the great success of her New York salon and expanding cosmetics line, Arden branched out into the destination spa business by opening a "beauty spa" in Maine in 1934 where women would pay more than $500 to spend a week losing weight, soaking in luxurious bath salts and trying out the latest lotions, makeup and beauty treatments. But it was her Red Door Salons in cities around the world that even through the Depression allowed Elizabeth Arden to successfully manage to keep women beautiful and pampered, no matter what the cost.

Today there are 31 Elizabeth Arden Red Door Spas and Resorts across the United States.

A Modern Day Spa Icon

Building on the achievements of her predecessor, Noelle de Caprio, founder of Noelle the Day Spa in Stamford, Connecticut in 1972, is also acclaimed as the founder of the modern Day Spa movement. She started by adding water-based treatments, specialized facials, massages and body treatments to her salon menu and, through hard work and charismatic personality, set an industry benchmark that has served as a beacon and catalyst for countless beauty industry professionals with a similar desire to provide more than just a few beauty treatments to their clients.

Her vision and dedication were truly inspirational, as was her generosity of spirit. Prior to her death in 1998 from a cancer that she had survived for over 14 years, Noelle had already taken her spa to the next level – wellness. Had she lived, she would be proud, I'm sure, to see how day spas across the continent, in ever-increasing numbers, have followed her example.

While some beauty and hair salons offer "spa" services, often they are tucked into a corner of the facility in order to justify using the word spa in their names.

Be sure to check whether the spa area is separate from the hair and nail/makeup area, as the two have different energy levels, including noise levels, which can impact the quiet enjoyment of your spa time.

On the other hand, with the advent of social networking, expect to find more spas integrating social areas where guests can mingle, check messages, interact and just hang out. In fact, many spas have already added spa parties and other opportunities for friends to come together in a more upbeat atmosphere, tuning in to the social aspect of spa as a place where like-minded individuals can enjoy each other's company in a safe and fun way.

Spas located in city hotels often exhibit all the characteristics of a day spa, as do some spas found in clubs and fitness facilities, reaching out to local guests and members to fill their appointment books, enhance their images and allow them to operate more profitably.

Go online or request a spa's brochure and start comparing the menus of different spas. You might be surprised to find that many of today's day spas sport treatment menus that rival those of even the most sophisticated resort and destination spas. Consequently, day spas provide spa goers with a perfect opportunity to continue their spa regimens locally between visits at their favourite "stay spas."

But please keep in mind that a huge treatment menu does not always equal a superlative spa experience. Many spas are trimming their menus and "getting back to basics" with a renewed emphasis on the professionalism and competence of their staff, augmented by superior customer service – so don't reject a spa just because it doesn't have, for instance, a couple's room or a Vichy shower.

Resort/Hotel Spas

It's difficult to find a Forbes Guide four-star or AAA four-diamond resort hotel in North America that doesn't include a spa, particularly in newer properties. The spa has become another major amenity within a hotel, similar to restaurants, meeting rooms, golf and other activities, and can vary in size from a few thousand square feet to over 50,000 square feet. What should you look for? Basically a spa in a hotel or resort should offer a full complement of services and treatments, including facials, nail care, massage and body treatments. Resort/hotels should generally offer at least a few spa-type low-cal items on their restaurant menus, as well. So, in regard to the question posed at the beginning of the chapter, the answer is no – a couple of massages offered in-room or around the pool area do not constitute a hotel spa no matter how the hotel, resort or inn tries to package them.

Interestingly, the addition of a spa to a hotel or resort's amenities can actually alter the overall ambience and atmosphere of the property – especially when the spa incorporates wellness programming and spa cuisine along with its regular services and treatments. In many resorts, it's not at all unusual to see guests walking about in robes or to find elements of the spa featured throughout the hotel. It depends upon how heavily the hotel chooses to incorporate the "relax, revitalize and rejuvenate" aspects of spa into its overall philosophy and culture.

A Quick Tip

It's always a good idea to book treatments well in advance of your hotel or resort stay rather than trusting to the availability of appointments once you arrive. Their spas tend to book up quickly, particularly on Fridays and Saturdays, and you don't want to miss that relaxing massage coming off the plane!

Resort spas are a perfect way for couples to learn the "ins and outs" of spa going in a relaxed atmosphere. Look for spas that feature couples treatments and use images of both men and women in their brochures and websites.

Destination Spas

A destination spa is a facility dedicated 100% to health, wellness, lifestyle and other spa-related activities. This includes its programming, which can be extensive, food chosen for its nutritive value and

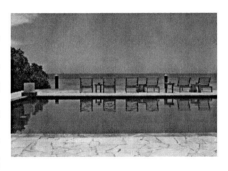

its accommodations. Stays are generally for a week or several days in order to successfully implement often highly intensive programs for weight loss; exercise, including hiking, kayaking, golf, tennis and other outdoor activities; healthy sleep; smoking cessation; or life enrichment programs and creative activities such as cooking classes, music appreciation, art, dance and other more esoteric topics presented by guest lecturers drawn from different walks of life. Take a look at Miraval, Canyon Ranch or Rancho La Puerta to get an idea of the depth and variety of the programs you'll find. Many destination spas also offer meeting space for companies and groups seeking to incorporate a spa-oriented schedule of activities into their meetings.

There are destination spas around the world that specialize in specific aspects of wellness and some that are purely luxurious, catering to relaxation and de-stressing. Many are all-inclusive with one price that includes accommodations, food and all activities except for a la carte spa services. They come in all shapes and sizes, but nearly all are dedicated to providing an enlightening, nurturing, relaxing and uplifting experience.

In many cases, it's becoming harder to differentiate between resort and destination spas because so many resort hotels exhibit many of the characteristics found in destination spas and vice versa. To better understand the differences, have a look at the Destination Spa Group with its stable full of North America's top destination spas catering to every possible desired personal outcome, not to mention great blogs and contributors.

Choosing a destination spa over a resort spa could depend upon how concerned you are with achieving one of the specific personal goals mentioned above. Or perhaps you are simply looking for a healthy environment where like-minded individuals gather to experience renewal of body, mind and spirit. One thing is for sure, if you're a single traveler, you'll find the camaraderie in destination spas ideal.

Mineral Springs Spas

If you live anywhere near a mineral springs spa, you're lucky! Mineral springs' waters, whether hot, cold or from the sea, have been healing and relaxing humans literally from the dawn of time and are enjoying a resurgence today as people look for stress-busting alternatives to drug store remedies. Depending on their chemical composition they can help alleviate a wide spectrum of 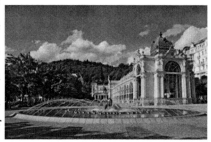 ailments, so it's no wonder that people are still drawn to them, even though many are fairly simple bathhouses or located in remote areas.

As of 2010, the International Spa Association reported 60 mineral springs spas in its 2010 U.S. Spa Industry Study — not that many when you consider that the U.S. has over 20,000 spas. In Europe, however, it's a different story with its rich history of therapeutic bathing traditions in countries like France, Germany, England, Belgium, the Czech Republic, Italy, Croatia, Romania and Austria. To this day, some of the most memorable water experiences you can imagine can be found in public mineral or warm springs bathhouses in cities like Bath, England; Spa, Belgium; Prague, Czech Republic; Budapest, Hungary or Baden-Baden, Germany.

Glen Ivy Hot Springs in Corona, California, is a wonderful example of the American mineral springs tradition. Nicknamed Club Mud for the rich, red clay mixed with the spring's mineral waters that guests have been smearing on themselves and each other for years, Glen Ivy has maintained its bath houses for a century and a half and has continuously reinvented itself in keeping with the changing times.

Other Relevant (Sub) Categories

Airport Spas

Few major airports in North America or Europe haven't got a "spa" or massage kiosk where you can while away the hours between flights or grab a quick fix for hands or body. Look for menus limited to basic face, nail and massage treatments suited to the energy of those travelers who have the time to drop in. Are these really spas? It's hard to manage the fluctuating and often crazy, wild energy of their clientele, yet many do it masterfully. As far as I'm concerned, when there are flight delays, having a quick treatment before boarding my plane leaves me feeling much more rested and alert when I arrive at my destination.

Cruise Ship Spas

Today, top spa brands such as Canyon Ranch, Six Senses or Elemis are represented on all the major cruise lines. They offer most of the treatments and services you would find in a shore spa operation, including a full range of facials, nail services, body treatments, signature treatments and fitness activities. Many companies like Celebrity Cruises encourage their guests to book appointments well in advance to avoid a disappointing lack of availability once on board. Cruise ship spas are comparable to resort spas since their guests, away from the pressures of their day-to-day lives, tend to be in a more relaxed frame of mind and apt to take advantage of all that the spa has to offer.

Hammams

One type of day spa, the hammam, is gaining in popularity in North America. What can you expect to find at a hammam? A perfect example is Ten Spa in Winnipeg, Manitoba. After showering, followed by a cup of Turkish tea, you enter the salting area, sit on a warm bench and apply a warm aromatic salt to yourself in order to begin perspiring and start your cleanse. In 10-15 minutes, after being rinsed off by your guide, you are escorted to the communal heated marble platform where you relax for another 30-60 minutes, pausing to pour hot, warm, cool or cold water over yourself. Depending on what you have booked, you might also receive a foot and scalp massage. This is followed by a traditional head-to-toe olive oil soap scrub-down, provided in a private treatment room. A rose oil massage afterwards is optional and the whole thing ends with a relaxing beverage post-treatment. Sounds divine? It is!

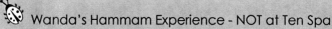 **Wanda's Hammam Experience - NOT at Ten Spa**

My first visit to a hammam was interesting, embarrassing and revitalizing. I had heard of hammams and was curious – then a chance encounter on the golf course with a gentleman who raved about a local hammam prompted me to finally make a reservation.

As I'm a bit shy and very self-conscious, I inquired during the reservation process about the "modesty" allowed during the treatment. It's rather important that I have the option to keep my private parts under cover throughout; I dislike having to disrobe in a public change room! After being assured that yes, draping protocols are recognized, I was quite happy to embark on the road to experience a hammam and gommage treatment.

Upon arrival, I was given a wrap to change into. While rather thin fabric, it was generous in size so I didn't feel exposed. I then was introduced to my therapist who led me to the treatment area, where I was instructed to remove my

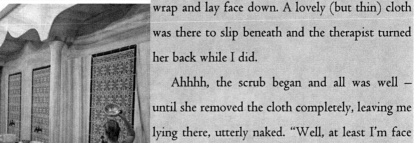

wrap and lay face down. A lovely (but thin) cloth was there to slip beneath and the therapist turned her back while I did.

Ahhhh, the scrub began and all was well – until she removed the cloth completely, leaving me lying there, utterly naked. "Well, at least I'm face down," I thought. Until minutes later when she requested I turn over. I was expecting she would have the draping cloth in front of her so I could roll over privately, before she placed the cloth over me so I wasn't exposed. No......she stood there impatiently waiting for me, no draping cloth in sight. I reluctantly turned over, silently praying the cloth would miraculously reappear. It didn't. I lay there naked, exposed, embarrassed and somewhat cold while she completed the treatment. While the exfoliation was lovely, it was hard to enjoy it as all I could think about was having my private parts and "wobbly bits" so fully exposed to a stranger.

When the scrub was complete, I was instructed to stand and face the wall to rinse off the exfoliant. The wall was a lovely slate tile, but I barely noticed, as I was still naked! I waited anxiously, expecting a gentle warm rinse – similar to a Vichy shower. Instead, I was hit with a strong spray of water from a hose held by my therapist. Rather than a relaxing, soothing water treatment, I felt more like I was standing naked against a prison wall while being hosed down for body lice.

"Spread your legs; lift your arms," – the indignity continued. And then the finale – "Turn around." Yup. Standing buck naked, shivering, facing a stranger who diligently hosed me down from head to toe. I felt like it lasted an eternity as my face flushed to a vibrant shade of magenta. Though I was hideously uncomfortable for much of the treatment, my skin was silky and smooth, and on the way home I was able to laugh about the day and my own inhibitions.

Much of my discomfort would have been easily avoided had I been advised upon booking that I would, in fact, be naked and exposed for a large portion of the treatment. As with many such experiences, it comes down to properly managing expectations.

- Wanda Love, Spa Adventurer and
Principal, Button Media Group

Nail Spas

So what is the difference between a nail salon and a nail spa? Nail spas are trending towards wellness, with some even adding podiatrists to deal with foot-related health issues. For instance, in the elegant surroundings of Isle PediSpa in Houston Texas, you are soothed by serene music and enveloped in aromatherapy scents while enjoying therapeutic foot and hand care as you sip sparkling water or an aromatic tea. Your safety is also a priority and all equipment is carefully sterilized or sanitized. That's not to say that a nail salon doesn't adhere to strict sanitation protocols, but the atmosphere tends to be a whole lot different, with less emphasis on mind, body and spirit and more on just getting your nails done and you on your way.

A Bit About Associations

Associations like the International Spa Association (ISPA) and Spa Industry Association of Canada (SIAC), formerly Leading Spas of Canada, advocate high standards of professionalism for their members from all of the above categories. They are a sure bet for finding a spa where you will receive treatments, services and programs provided by skilled and competent staff in a safe environment.

The North American spa industry is relatively new and largely unregulated. From the national level down to the local level in both the U.S. and Canada, the only spa-oriented regulations and guidelines in most jurisdictions are concerned with general sanitation and health safety.

In response, over a decade ago the International Spa Association and the Spa Industry Association of Canada each mandated a reasonable, yet comprehensive, set of Standards and Practices applicable to spas of every type to foster the overall professionalism of the industry, to ensure the quality of the Spa Experience in member spas and for the safety and protection of the general public in both countries. Their members pledge to uphold these Standards and Practices as well as a very specific code of ethics.

The Spa Industry Association of Canada has taken it a step further through a Quality Assurance program of participating spas, with bi-annual assessments conducted by an independent third-party that gives the public the confidence that program members meet or exceed SIAC's published Standards and Practices.

In terms of Quality Assurance, there are other organizations equally dedicated to upholding high standards of professionalism within the industry. For instance, SpaQuality LLC has been steadily raising the awareness of quality in spas and providing tools to improve quality systems in spas worldwide since 2004.

In addition, in both ISPA and SIAC, the products and services provided by member companies and purveyors to the spa industry (such as skin care, cosmeceutical and equipment companies) must also meet a set of standards comparable to those set for spas.

This is not to imply that spas or manufacturers that are not association members are necessarily inferior. Many choose not to belong for a variety of reasons, from the cost of dues to perhaps a lack of understanding of the value of a membership. However, those that do are willing to pay sometimes high annual dues or fees in order to join with other professionals to learn as much as they can, share the knowledge that they have with their contemporaries and work together to further the spa industry wherever they may be.

In other words, don't hesitate to go online to the association websites at the end of this book and feel more confident about that spa down the street that displays a recognized spa association decal on its door, on its website or in the spa itself.

Authenticity and the Spa Experience

Over the years, spa consumers have become increasingly sophisticated and very savvy, seeking services and products that are original, honest and real. They want to "experience" service at all levels and want to see results – expectations that, not surprisingly, are mirrored in the non-spa going public, as well.

At first a trend, authenticity in the spa is now commonly found in the textiles, furnishings and design elements that reflect the environment in which the spa is located. It exists in the music and scents; in the treatment products that make use of indigenous plants, muds and seaweeds and in the treatments themselves. So much so, in fact, that authenticity is now the norm and is expected and sought after by consumers worldwide.

A Perfect Example

In contrast to such beautiful destinations as Bali, Tahiti and other exotic places, consider Hills Health Ranch in 108 Mile House, British Columbia. It doesn't get much more authentic than this. Pat and Juanita Corbett started the health resort/destination spa in 1985 as a result of personal health issues that had raised their awareness of their need for a change to a healthier lifestyle. Putting their money where their mouths were, they started The Hills on 20,000 acres of beautiful British Columbia backcountry as a place where people could come to kick-start their lives in a healthier direction. Since then, tens of thousands have travelled to this rustically beautiful destination spa to shed pounds, quit smoking, ride horses, cross-country ski, eat (yes, fabulous food!) and partake in a wide variety of activities with a wellness focus.

It's a perfect combination of spa and an old-fashioned dude ranch, replete with hayrides and sing-alongs. Its sixteen treatment rooms feature treatments for face and body – some using Rose Hip Oil made from rose hips gathered in the surrounding hills and cold-pressed on-site in equipment imported from Germany.

Miles of riding/cross country ski trails trace the countryside, making this a full-on active year round destination. Yet The Hills is quite a bit more sophisticated than you might at first think, since it has long been a leader in nutritional counselling, with their highly qualified nutritionists, and fitness training, with yoga, Pilates and Aquafit trainers/instructors, and on-staff Medical Doctors. The "hype" matches, and is more often than not surpassed by, the quality and professionalism of their services and products. A well-appointed fitness centre and exercise pool round out the many other spa amenities.

The Corbett's and their staff are extraordinary examples of "walking the talk." Their passion and dedication to providing their guests with the tools for wellness and a healthier lifestyle have made them icons of the spa industry and the recipients of numerous awards, most recently the International Spa Association's 2009 award for Dedicated Contributor.

Authenticity? It's when you're walking along a path between the spa and your A-frame cabin deep in thought and come across a horse sauntering along, without saddle, bridle or tack of any kind, on its way to the lower pasture for the night. You look around, see another, then another, until they've all made their way, slowly ambling past in the same direction, and then feel a keen sense of utter joy for having been the recipient of such a momentous experience.

Authenticity isn't always the case, however. In an effort to lure clients in their doors, some spas make promises they can't keep, such as promoting anti-aging treatments with instant, dramatic results or "indigenous" products and treatments that are not in the least relevant to the spa's location or environment. The good news is that you, the consumer, are the ultimate arbiter. Just keep in mind that when you do find a spa that isn't keeping it real, it's a reflection on the ethics and business practices of the owner, not the entire spa industry.

Interesting International Indigenous Treatments

Alpine Wellness	Hopi Ear Candling
Australian Aboriginal	Hungarian Mud
Balinese Lulur	Indian Head Massage
Brazilian Wax	Italian Fango
British Health Farm	Japanese Shiatsu
Mexican Temescal	Chinese Acupuncture
Philippine Hilot	Dead Sea Salt Scrub
Russian Steam	Egyptian Oils
Scottish Shower	French Thalassotherapy
Swiss Shower	Finnish Sauna
Thai Massage	Turkish Hammam
Hawaiian Lomi Lomi	Canadian Maple Sugar Scrub

From Susie Ellis' "International Language of Spa"

On another note, in addition to indigenous treatments, the general public's increased sensitivity to environmental issues has led to consumer demand for eco-friendly and organic spa treatments and products. In fact, by 2009, demand for eco and organic had outpaced the demand for indigenous treatments,[1] leading to a proliferation of organic skin care lines with many of the major, more established skin care companies adding organic products to their lines or adopting a more "organic" look.

  From Sea to Thee

Diane Bernard, affectionately known on Vancouver Island, British Columbia, as the Seaweed Lady, harvests kelp and seaweeds from some of the over 150 species of seaweeds growing in the cold, pristine coastal waters off Vancouver Island. The resulting organic skin care line, Seaflora, features seaweed/algae products that are pure and unadulterated and used by many spas on the Island and across Canada and the U.S.

An outing with Diane is an adventure – while wading along the shore in gum boots, not only do you learn about the various kelp and seaweeds that grow along the Pacific Coast, you can touch and taste them as well!

The Word Spa as a Marketing Tool

Look around and you're bound to see the word often grossly misused in reference to products and commodities. What is it about the word that conveys such an image of health, quality and/or exclusivity? It can be found on drug store shelves, in grocery store aisles, salons, department stores and is a favourite word of the media.

Perhaps the answer lies in the fact that spa embodies lifestyle choices in a way that no other concept can. It speaks to our desire for simplicity, purity and serenity in our mad and hectic world.

What's in Store?

As spas continue to evolve, look for an increasing emphasis on health and wellness both in day and stay spas. And you'll find spa services being introduced on trains, ferries and other places where individuals have a few extra moments to take advantage of them.

Spa communities will spring up everywhere, while many retirement communities will add spa-related services as part of their programs. With an emphasis on wellness and prevention, expect their residents to be more vigorous well into advanced old age than elsewhere.

The social aspect of spa will be magnified as you are given more opportunities to interact both with other spa guests or your personal tablet, phone or other assorted equipment in a safe, relaxed atmosphere. And more and more apps will enable you to find the spa experience you're looking for.

Sustainability will continue to find increasing resonance within the spa community, combined with a greater appreciation of our inter-relatedness with our physical and spiritual environments. Check out greenspanetwork.org or ecospas.com to gain a greater understanding of the steps spas are taking to stay in balance and harmony with the environment.

You will be able to give the gift of spa more easily and in a much more personalized way than before with digital gifting – a trend that will soon replace plastic cards – as more and more spas jump on the bandwagon.

In summary, although spas continue to evolve in step with societal changes, they will remain havens where people can go to reaffirm their humanity in terms of their physical, spiritual and emotional wellbeing.

Chapter 2   How to Choose the Right Spa for You

Choosing the right spa is a bit like choosing a restaurant. First you have to decide what you're in the mood for and then how much you want to spend. After that, everything else sort of falls into place – well, almost!

We'll take a look at five clues to finding the right spa for you, what spa pricing says about the spa and the various ways to learn about spas in your area, especially through social media.

First, a Bit About a Spa's Ambience

Spas come in all shapes and sizes, and in all styles and decors. In one, you'll find a Zen-like atmosphere of tranquility and calm; in another, marble, columns and draperies combine to create a European flavour; while in the next, a modern, neutral decor gives off strong uni-sex vibes. Some spas spend hundreds of thousands, even millions, of dollars to create an unforgettable space while others are fortunate enough to be able to offer an exquisite, oceanside experience that doesn't cost a cent to provide.

What is their common denominator? To experience spa is to engage all five of your senses – something that should be immediately apparent in the physical surroundings of any spa from the moment you enter.

Spa and the Five Senses

Everything in a spa should appeal to each of the five senses: smell, taste, hearing, sight and touch. These elements should be integrated in such a way that they work together to impart a state of relaxation and ease; to lower your stress levels and heighten your appreciation of the treatments and services you receive.

🌸   *Smell*

Since your sense of smell can have such an impact on your emotions and sense of wellbeing, especially when combined with taste, smells can set the stage for the appreciation – or the lack thereof – of your spa experience. Many spas employ aromatherapy scents to underscore their themes and are keenly aware of the importance of appealing to their guest's olfactory systems with pleasant herbal and/or floral aromas. Personally, I prefer a fresh, neutral scent, but that's just me.

In no case should you smell hair or nail chemicals or other unpleasant odours. Ventilation in those areas should be adequate to remove them.

❦ Taste

Look for a pitcher of water or a tea urn sitting on a sideboard in the reception area or lounge, even in some of the smaller day spas. Lemons, cucumbers or limes are often added to the water to refresh your palate. Or a cup of soothing herbal tea or fresh fruit may be offered to relax you and put you in a spa state of mind.

❦ Hearing

Music is soothing and low key in the spa area. If the spa incorporates hair care, often combined with nail care, you can expect to hear more upbeat music, but that music should not compete with the overall calm and serene atmosphere of the rest of the spa. In the treatment rooms, particularly when you have a choice of music, the walls and doors should be soundproof to prevent the wash of outside noises and music from the corridors from interfering.

This is a pet peeve of mine and one which can ruin the experience for me — two different music beats happening at once, footsteps clacking along the corridor or voices raised as people pass by while I'm in a treatment. To combat this, some spas offer ear pods, along with a selection of soothing music.

❦ Sight

Whether hundreds of thousands or simply a few thousand dollars have been spent on interior design, it is the spa's meticulous attention to detail that determines its overall positive impact.

Looking around, what do you see? When you step up to the reception desk, a messy work surface might be a clue that perhaps not all is as it should be. Product displays and makeup stands should be clean and uncluttered; furniture and equipment must be in good repair and there should be an overall sense of well-kept tidiness. Bits and pieces of equipment not in use should be stored out of your sight — not on tops of cabinets or under tables.

Lighting is also important in creating a pleasing ambience. Many spas pay careful attention to their choice of lighting, thereby creating their desired atmosphere and feel.

✦ Touch

Deep comfortable seating, a soft, plush robe, the feel of a duvet placed over you during your facial or a warmed pad laid over your back and shoulders to relax you before they are massaged enhance the experience. A room too cold, especially during a wet body treatment, can cause muscles to tense up, leaving you wondering when the ordeal will finally be over. Rough towels and linens aren't any fun either!

In a well-run spa all these points will have been gladly addressed for your safety, comfort and enjoyment and will be so well done that you would only notice if they hadn't.

As far as furnishings, size and design are concerned, regardless of where you are, within your own community or as you travel, you will almost certainly find one that appeals to your personal sense of style and taste.

Five Clues to Choosing the Right Spa for You

When you're looking for just the right spa, there are five things to keep in mind to help make the search a little easier: purpose, value, ambience, location and qualifications.

I. Purpose.

The type of treatment you want (or need) will help narrow down your choice.

Example: would you look for a waxing expert in a spa that specializes in anti-aging treatments? While not mutually exclusive, a good day spa is probably your best bet for the first and a medical spa for the latter. So you'll want to do your homework. Ask around and compare menus online whether in your community or while travelling.

2. Value.

It is generally agreed that the price of a treatment in relation to its perceived level of performance and quality creates the value of the overall experience, with ambience, location and qualifications entering into the equation, as well.

Example: if you visit a spa in a high-end resort and receive a rushed and impersonal (but expensive) treatment, no matter how beautifully furnished the spa, your perception of its value will invariably suffer as a result.

Once you have completed your treatment, only you will be able to judge whether you have received the value you had anticipated. But be fair. The old adage, "You get what you pay for," holds true in the spa world as well.

3. Ambience.

A great many things enter into a spa's ambience – its character and atmosphere – and it really is up to you to decide what will make you happy.

Example: perhaps beautiful change rooms, a well-stocked retail centre or water amenities like saunas, steam rooms or pool aren't important to you at the moment – maybe a small spa in a strip mall is exactly what you're looking for. Make a list of the spas that interest you; take a few hours and visit them to see how they make you feel.

4. Location.

Where you live, your climate and the number of spas near you will heavily influence your choice of spa. The same goes for your travel destinations.

Example: in a fairly small town you might have relatively few spas to choose from, while in a larger city the option of an up-scale urban hotel/day spa instead of a little day spa around the corner is not unusual. Fortunately, there are thousands of spas worldwide that can provide the type of experience you seek.

5. Qualifications.

The most valuable resource a spa has is its team of professionals. Opt only for those spas with well-trained, courteous and helpful staff, regardless of the treatment.

Example: good spas demand that their therapists, estheticians and nail techs have either passed state or provincial licensing (if required) or have graduated from accredited cosmetology and massage schools. It's your right to check.

In terms of the spa's physical qualifications, hygiene and cleanliness are equally important. You don't want to risk infection from improperly cleaned implements or unsanitary equipment.

Tuck these clues into the back of your mind for a more intelligent approach to narrowing down the choices you face with the multitude of spa options available today.

Where to Find the Right Spa for You

When choosing a local spa, your best bet is the advice and recommendations of your friends and family — those most likely to let you know whether a particular spa offers superior and consistent service. In fact, word of mouth remains the number one way in which consumers find a reliable spa.

Alternatively, spas tend to make frequent use of local broadcast media to get their word out by running contests or advertising on local radio and television stations. If your newspaper has an annual "Best of City," see which spas made it, as well as being on the lookout for spa ads in them – whether print or online.

The "Reader's Choice" annual awards found at Spa Magazine, Condé Nast Traveler Magazine, Travel and Leisure Magazine, Spas of America, SpaFinder, Forbes and elsewhere showcase top spas from around the world. Study the winners' websites for examples of creative and beautifully crafted treatment menus that will help you better understand what makes a spa exceptional, and if there's one near you, go have a look.

If you're going on vacation and think you might want to have a few quality spa treatments, start with finding a spa in your destination of choice and then book the hotel, inn or resort it's in. There are a number of top-notch spa booking and travel services, like www.spafinder.com, www.spasofamerica.com and www.discoverspas.com that are listed at the end of the book to help you decide. Just be sure to also book your spa treatment at the same time you book your room!

Spa brands are on the rise. Well, actually, many have been around for quite a while, like Bliss Spas, Six Senses, Red Door Spas, Away Spas, Willow Stream and others, but more and more, you will find different, less well-known multi-location spa brands appearing somewhere near you. On the whole, in order to be part of the brand "family," these spas have to comply with the standards and requirements that each particular brand has established in order to capture its share of the spa going market. So, when you hear of one in your area, use the Five Clues to Finding the Right Spa for You to see if it's something you'd be interested in.

And don't forget to look into the member spas of the International Spa Association or Spa Industry Association of Canada. Their reputable day and stay spa members pledge to uphold their association's Standards and Practices, promising the safety and quality of your spa experience wherever it may be.

You'll find customer feedback on a wide variety of sites, from Spa Finder to Yelp. But unless there are several opinions, allowing you to weigh the often very positive or negative comments expressed, take them with a grain of salt, hmm?

Many urban hotels have lovely spas and perhaps you would prefer that particular ambience to a spa in a strip mall. If you've found a spa you like but aren't sure, inquire with your local Better Business Bureau. In any case, do some online comparative shopping and get a feel for the place through its website.

But be a little careful, too. For instance, if you're looking for laser hair removal or microdermabrasion treatments, I suggest that you choose a medical spa with medically supervised staff. And only an MD should administer Botox® and fillers. I like to err on the side of caution.

What Pricing Says About a Spa

Do you expect the same level of service and quality of food at a McDonalds that you do in a fine dining establishment? Of course not. Yet many people question why they should pay $125 for an hour's massage at a Willow Stream spa when they can find one for $49 at a Massage Envy location. The answer is that although both employ licensed massage therapists and provide good treatments, at Massage Envy you won't find the plush robes, relaxation areas, plunge pools, well-appointed change/locker areas or the variety of treatments and services that you would at a Willow Stream spa. There's a world of difference between the two and each fills a distinct market niche, providing the consumer with clear-cut choices, and without trying to be all things to all people.

It's important to remember that spas are businesses, too. Your geographical area, the size or type of spa and the number of spas in competition with each other are additional factors that relate to price. Moreover, spas are intensively service-oriented – their most precious resource is their staff – but well-trained staff means higher labour costs that are inevitably reflected in their treatment prices.

Lastly, consider that many of the specialized products used in spa treatments are of a very high quality and very intensive in their effectiveness. They're made from often quite unique ingredients and consequently cost a lot to create or manufacture. Even though spa owners strive to keep down the cost of their treatments, in order to maximize results for their guests, most owners are unwilling to forgo using these quality products, adding to the prices of their treatments as a result.

> Ask about your service provider's credentials. Price can often be indicative of the level of training, quality and professionalism of the spa's staff.

The Importance of Social Media

Spas of every type are now offering specials that range from a treatment with a gift or spa product thrown in to reduced prices on selected treatments and services. They are normally posted on their web sites, Facebook or Twitter, so be sure to look out for them. You can find some wonderful promotions and special offerings.

❦ *Facebook*

Many spas have a Facebook page and use it to communicate with guests and clients in a variety of ways: posting specials, describing their treatments, talking about new product lines and keeping things fresh and current. It is now an integral part of many spas' overall marketing strategies.

❦ *Twitter*

Look for great deals at spas that tweet their specials to fill up their appointment books. You might find a tweet that announces "two spots available this afternoon for a facial for $20" or something similar – some really sweet deals. Spas and spa bloggers also tweet information or stories about the newest treatments, products and happenings in the world of spa, so be sure to follow once you've found one you like.

* *Online Deal Sites*

Groupon, Living Social, Spa Week, Spa Rah Rah, Wahanda, Rue La La and others consistently offer great, limited time deals on spas and are fairly well represented in the medium to large urban centres. Exercise caution, though. Sites like Groupon that are not specifically spa-oriented will feature any spa that wants to use them as a marketing tool. This is not to discredit Groupon, rather to say that before you buy a coupon, go online to the spa's website and get a feel for it (also check your local Better Business Bureau). The spa's presence on Groupon says nothing about the spa's quality.

* *SEO and Applications*

Using search engines to find spas in your area is still one of the most effective methods available. Nearly every spa, whether large or small, has a website. Or perhaps you've found a brand of facial care on your travels that really appeals to you. Look on the product line's website to find a spa location near you that carries it. By the way, this is an especially good way to find a reputable medical spa or provider for Botox® injections.

As for applications, a good example is Massage Envy's that allows you to pinpoint the part of your body that needs attention and the amount of pressure you would prefer, giving your therapist specific information about you before you even start your treatment. Canyon Ranch offers fitness and healthy eating apps. And the list of spa apps is growing as more and more spas jump on the spa app bandwagon to allow even greater customization of your spa experience.

* *Blogs*

Many spas, spa associations, spa magazines, spa-related websites and spa-going individuals feature highly informative, but sometimes very opinionated blogs. While most contain valid information and observations, not all do. An old adage that states, "paper is tolerant," applies equally to the web. When you find a topic that interests you or you read a blog that sounds a little biased one way or the other, don't hesitate to look at other websites on the subject and compare.

Finding a spa today – one that will meet and fulfill your needs and expectations – has never been easier. Do your homework and reap the benefits of regular visits to the spa!

Chapter 3   Getting the Most Out of Your Spa Time

So, you've decided to put your toe in the proverbial water and make an appointment for your very first facial. Congratulations!

But wait…. you're a little shy about calling and showing the receptionist that you haven't got a clue as to what's involved in their *basic* facial – not to mention the difference between the aquamarine or lymphatic facial described in the menu you just finished perusing online. OK, so you also looked at a couple of YouTube videos on the subject, but is that how this spa does things?

Rather than eagerly looking forward to your visit, there's just the tiniest bit of trepidation niggling at the back of your mind. Not a very auspicious start to your spa journey at all!

Sometimes we (in the spa industry) forget how confusing a lot of our jargon is to the average non-spa goer when we describe the various treatments on our spa menus. Terms like alpha-hydroxy peels, lymph drainage, hydrating infusions or anti-free radical masks are a bit overwhelming and intimidating even to many who have been to a spa more than once.

My guess is that you'd appreciate having something of a basic yardstick with which to measure your spa visit, something that would raise your comfort level. Basics that give you the assurance that the prices and the overall professionalism of the spa are in line as well.

Top 10 Ways to Make the Most of your Spa Experience

Following are a number of best practices that should be the cornerstone of any spa operation, whether day or stay spa. Some have to do with how you are perceived and treated as their guest and others have to do with your safety while in their spa environment. Still others are steps you can take to ensure that that your time in the spa provides you with the best experience possible – and the greatest benefits.

First Contact

I. Booking Your Appointment

The Reception Desk is the hub of any well-run spa, just as it is in a hotel or doctor's office, because the efficiency and effectiveness of the entire spa operation – keeping things on time, accurate information gathering, dealing with customers before and after their treatments, etc. – depends on the person(s) sitting behind that desk.

Thank goodness for online booking, Facebook and other social media sources, but when you have questions, especially if this is the first time you're visiting the spa, there's nothing like having a live voice on the phone to query.

Your point of contact for booking your appointment should be well-trained and in her position long enough to have experienced a few treatments (especially the signature services) in order to be able to describe them effectively to you. If she can't, say that you're more than happy to wait while she finds out.

Let her know whether you prefer a male or female therapist, especially for a massage or body treatment. For instance, if I'm looking for a firmer massage, I'll often request a male therapist, secure in the knowledge that my modesty is safe because of proper draping techniques.

Are you pregnant? Do you have any significant medical problems, such as heart, high blood pressure or thyroid, that need to be considered? You might want to bring that up now even though you'll be filling out a guest history form when you arrive. Although some spas have staff that specialize in treatments for specific conditions, to be fair, it just makes good sense to give them advance notice rather than assuming that your particular issue can be handled easily.

Your booking agent will also confirm your contact information, and if you should ask for details, will let you know about taxes, extra charges, if any, or extra amenities that you can make use of while at the spa (like bathing pools, steam rooms, saunas, exercise equipment, etc.).

And when you arrive? For me, my visit begins on a high when the receptionist greets me with warmth and courtesy. Is this old-fashioned? Maybe so, but it sure can put me at my ease, especially when visiting a spa for the first time – or any time, for that matter!

2.   Cancelling or Rescheduling an Appointment

In addition to informing you of the spa's cancellation policy, generally 24 to 48 hours in advance, you could be asked to give a credit card number to secure your appointment (and some spas even ask for payment for part or all of your appointment in advance). If a cancellation policy seems unfair, look at it from the spa's perspective – not only are they losing the revenue that you would generate, but they have tied up a treatment room that most likely can't be filled that day. They've also probably had to turn away business for your time slot, especially when they're busy.

Usually the day before, the spa will call or email a reminder of your visit. This is something I really appreciate, because I get so busy sometimes that I neglect to look at my calendar.

Before Your Arrival

3.   Food, Drink and Shaving

Whether you're male or female, the only thing you'll want to drink before your treatment is a bit of water. Try to avoid food and dehydrating drinks – particularly alcoholic beverages – near your treatment time. If you're on vacation, schedule your appointment away from meal times to make sure you really enjoy yourself without suffering some sort of adverse reaction. Then, after your treatment, drink water and plenty of it to flush the toxins that are released during your treatment out of your body.

As for shaving (whether legs or other body parts), try not to do so immediately before a service, as your skin might become irritated and susceptible to infection. If it's unavoidable, advise your therapist so that she can use products that soothe the skin or prepare it appropriately for the treatment to follow. However, if you're a guy booking a facial, many spas will request that you shave just prior to your appointment.

4. Jewellery and Valuables

As for jewellery, you might want to leave your valuables at home – it's up to you. Since I generally have my watch and rings on all the time (and forget to leave them home!), I make it a point of leaving them locked in my locker in my purse or on a dish in the treatment room if changing there. Most spas do not assume liability for lost or stolen valuables, even from a locked locker, so I'm probably tempting fate – I know.

Now You've Arrived

5. Be On Time

You'll be asked to arrive a few minutes early, so do yourself and the spa a favour and make that at least 15 minutes in advance so that you can fill out any forms, change, stow your personal belongings and visit the rest room one more time before starting your treatment punctually. And don't forget to bring a bathing suit if you plan on taking a swim, steam or sauna beforehand and, obviously, you'll want to arrive even earlier if you do!

Many spas advise their guests that the minutes they're late will be subtracted from their treatment time. If this sounds harsh, remember that the treatment rooms are booked back to back in order to maximize the number of guests that can be seen on any given day. Being late, even a few minutes per treatment, can add up to a very late afternoon or evening for spa personnel. Being on time keeps their stress levels lower and allows them to maximize your enjoyment.

6. Guest History Forms

When you arrive, you'll be asked to take a seat and fill out the guest history form as completely and accurately as possible. It only takes a few minutes. This will alert your therapist to the products she should use, any medical problems you might have, the most suitable treatment to recommend and allow her to ask you more specific and targeted questions.

 A Bit About Guest History Forms

Some people consider this a real nuisance, but it can save both you *and* the spa a lot of headaches. By the way, if you're a regular at the spa, let them know if there have been any changes to your health history since the last visit, so that they can modify your information accordingly.

A Sorry Story

Not long after we had opened our spa in the early 90's, a mother and daughter came in for what was to be a girl's day out in preparation for a speech competition in which the seventeen-year-old daughter was to participate the following week. They had a couple of treatments, ending in a facial for each. One of the questions we didn't have on the Guest History form at that time was whether the individual used products containing Retinol (or similar). Given the girl's age and appearance, the esthetician didn't think to ask before agreeing to wax her cheeks and upper lips at the girl's request. It later turned out that she had been taking Retin-A for over a year (which can result in a thinning of the stratum corneum or outer layer of the skin with the result that waxing can "burn," tear or otherwise damage the skin).

You can guess the rest of the story. Though not badly affected (it looked like a bad sunburn), the results were very upsetting to the girl and her mother. Our spa was subsequently sued for the potential four-year scholarship that the girl could have won if she had looked and felt "normal." The esthetician was, of course, devastated and so were we all.

A hard lesson, to be sure, but it showed me early on just how important it is to gather as much complete and accurate information from the guest as possible.

I'm a little leery of spas that don't have at least a cursory form to fill out. Don't they care??

After you have filled out your guest history information, you'll be escorted to the change room and directed to go from there to either the lounge or a waiting area or you'll be asked to follow your therapist to your treatment room, if changing or disrobing there. This will probably be the first contact you will have with your therapist, so don't be hesitant or shy and try to establish a personal connection to that person before beginning your treatment.

In the Treatment Room

7. Cleanliness and Hygiene

Besides the obvious, like clean and uncluttered surfaces on floors, counters and cabinets, there are a number of practices that ensure that the spa has your health and safety at heart.

Top 10 Things to Keep on Your Spa Radar Screen

I. Your therapist should have on a neat and clean uniform or slacks and shirt (male or female). Nails should be trimmed and hair, if longer than chin length, tied back. Just as it is your obligation to the spa not to wear perfumes to an appointment, it's the therapist's responsibility to have a completely neutral smell – including cigarette odours or bad breath! And in the case of a cold, he or she should wear a mask.

2. Your therapist should thoroughly wash her hands before and after your treatment. It's even better if there is a sink in the room so that she can do it in

your presence - particularly in flu season when germs can be so easily transmitted through contact. And if she leaves the room, she should wash her hands each time she returns!

3.   Speaking of which, your therapist should wear disposable gloves whenever performing waxing, pedicures or for extractions during a facial. The gloves used are so thin that you barely notice them on your skin and will be discarded after your treatment. Though this might seem wasteful, it's for your mutual benefit and just plain good hygiene.

4.   A cardinal rule in the waxing room is that a fresh spatula must be used each time the therapist dips into the wax pot to apply wax to any part of your body. Why? The wax (usually vegetable based) doesn't get hot enough (only about 40 degrees Celsius) to kill bacteria or fungus and once the spatula comes in contact with your skin can transmit bacteria and viruses back into the wax if double dipped. Don't even think about the personal hygiene habits of the person who was in the room before you!

As for the paraffin wax used for hands and feet during a manicure or pedicure, when the appendage in question is dipped into the wax, some manufacturers claim that since the body temperature is around 15 degrees cooler than the wax, the wax immediately solidifies, encapsulating any bacteria or impurities on the skin and avoiding contamination of the wax. This, of course, assumes that the temperature of the wax is properly maintained at 130 degrees Fahrenheit or 54 degrees Celsius.

However, if the spa is observing good hygiene, the therapist will fill the wax into a plastic baggie and then have you place your hand or foot into it. You have no way of knowing whether the wax pot is operating properly, do you?

5. You can also count on the fact that a good spa, as a matter of course, disinfects slippers or flip flops between guests, provides fresh bath mats prior to each treatment and furnishes you with spanking clean towels and robes. Bed linens are also changed between appointments ensuring that everything is fresh for you.

6. As for disinfection, more and more spas are switching to autoclaves to thoroughly sterilize implements used in treatments. Though chemical disinfectants and sterilizers take care of most bacteria, fungi and viruses, not all kill spores, but autoclaves do. Conscientious use of hospital grade disinfectants is a further measure they take - especially for cleaning footbaths.

7. Speaking of which, all footbaths and jetted tubs (hydrotherapy tubs), whether they are self cleaning or not, must be cleaned with a disinfectant between clients. Look to make sure that this is the case. And don't worry, during your pedicure treatment, more often than not, at least one of the chairs will be prepped for the next guest, so you'll be able to see for yourself. If you have any concerns, please be sure to ask. Really – it's your health at stake!

8. Your spa should also use disposable nail files and buffers. In any case, implements and tools used more than once per guest must be disinfected. If you have any concerns, take your own implements with you, just in case.

9. Be sure to check bathroom sink and shower drains to make sure that they're free of "debris" and clean. With some of the other points above, you might be somewhat hesitant to ask, but clean restrooms and change rooms are a dead giveaway as to the levels of hygiene and cleanliness behind the scenes in the rest of the spa.

10. Make sure that you leave the change room/area the way you found it. Throw wet towels and your used robe into the appropriate containers. Same goes for flip flops or slippers. Keep in mind that not every spa has a full complement of personal amenities, so if there's something out of the ordinary you know you'll need after your treatment, either check with the booking agent to see whether it's furnished by the spa or bring it from home. If you do make use of the amenities they normally provide, such as shampoos and lotions, please replace them where they belong.

Give your locker one last check to make sure you haven't left anything behind. The next guest will appreciate it and the spa will love you.

It goes without saying that by maintaining good hygiene practices, in addition to protecting your health and ensuring your safety, your spa is making every effort for you to be able to relax and truly enjoy yourself.

8. Letting Go

Can you? Part from your cell phone for the length of your treatment? Most spas require that cell phones be turned off, although some, I think, allow their use because they want to respect their guests' need to stay connected and allow those who find it more stressful to be without their cells to keep them close at hand.

My take is that when you opt for a visit to a spa – even if it's for a maintenance service like a pedicure or manicure – there should be a certain rhythm and flow to your time there. You're supposed to be putting away the cares and worries of the outside world for a few minutes in order to center and rebalance yourself by staying in that flow. Your therapist also wants to be "in the moment" with you so that you both can make the most of your visit. Why spoil that by talking or texting during a treatment? Especially talking on your cell and expecting those around you to share your conversation!

9. Talking

For the most part, I prefer to be quiet, in the moment and use my time at the spa to relax, not chatting about — whatever. That's most important to me during a massage and I also get so relaxed during a pedicure that I've been known to fall asleep and drool. Ew!

On the other hand, from a professional standpoint, if the therapist needs to alert me to something during the treatment, I want her to do so. Especially during a facial. Then I want to know exactly what she's using on me and why as she moves through the various stages of the treatment. She can point out any number of things, from overly dry skin to rosacea and suggest the appropriate treatment. Nevertheless, some people find these suggestions a "hard sell" of the spa's skin care products and find it a huge negative. If that describes you, then simply ask your esthetician to wait until the end of the treatment to discuss them with you or say that you're not interested in purchasing at this time. That's perfectly all right.

In no case do the personal problems of the therapist have a place in the treatment room. How much you talk is up to you. If you don't want to, and the therapist keeps on talking, simply say something like, "Think I'm going to just be quiet and enjoy this now." She'll get the message and stop, don't worry. That way, you'll still be able to get the most out of the service and won't feel the need to complain at the end.

10. Spa Products – To Buy or Not to Buy?

Nearly every spa offers beauty products, including skin care and makeup, for you to purchase to enhance and maintain your regular skin care regimen at home. Whether you do or not is up to you. Look around and you might find a number of other things that make great hostess gifts or that would help you take the spa experience home – like music, journals, books, candles and whimsical objects you wouldn't find elsewhere.

If you find that the product that you've purchased doesn't work for you for some reason, you should be able to return it. Often the spa's return policy is posted on its website, but if not you might want to look into the spa's policy with the receptionist before making your purchase. Just remember to give the product a chance to prove its effectiveness, generally at least a couple of weeks, before returning it.

A Bit About Gratuities

Today, most spas include a tipping policy in their spa literature or online. If not, as a rule of thumb, tip just as you would in a restaurant for good service – 15% to 20% in North America. Some spas include an automatic service charge per treatment, especially for groups or multiple treatments. The service charge is made in lieu of (replaces) gratuities and it would be up to you to add a gratuity over and above that, if you feel the service has been superlative.

If you are visiting the spa on a gift certificate or Groupon-type "deal," be sure to ask at the desk whether the gift giver has included the gratuity, and tip appropriately if it's not!

Please note that tipping practices and service charges vary from country to country. If you're a seasoned globetrotter, you're aware of this, but if you're not, simply check with the spa receptionist. Don't be shy about it – your therapist will be most grateful, especially in countries where wages are low and people depend on gratuities to enhance their incomes. However, in some countries like Japan, a gratuity is considered insulting, so asking beforehand is always a good idea.

Are you feeling a little more confident about becoming part of the increasing number of men and women taking charge of their health and wellbeing by visiting a spa? Good! Read on for more useful information and tips on everything from men's treatments and medical spas to facials, massage and nail care. Remember, knowing what to expect is your key to an enjoyable and beneficial spa experience.

CODE OF CONDUCT

Your Rights and Responsibilities as a Spa Guest[1]

As a Spa Guest, it is your responsibility to:

1. Communicate your preferences, expectations and concerns;
2. Communicate complete and accurate health information and reasons for your visit;
3. Treat staff and other guests with courtesy and respect;
4. Use products, equipment and therapies as directed;
5. Engage in efforts to preserve the environment; and
6. Adhere to the spa's published policies and procedures.

As a Spa Guest, you have the right to:

7. A clean, safe and comfortable environment;
8. Stop a treatment at any time, for any reason;
9. Be treated with consideration, dignity and respect;
10. Confidential treatment of your disclosed health information;
11. Trained staff who respectfully conduct treatments according to treatment protocols and the spa's policies and procedures;
12. Ask questions about your spa experience; and
13. Information regarding staff training, licensing and certification.

[1] *Officially endorsed and prepared in partnership by:*
International Spa Association and Resort Hotel Association

Chapter 4   Macho, Macho Man

Let's start with you men. Have you been thinking about going to a spa? Maybe your best friend can't stop talking about the great massage he had, and it's enough to make you curious – but you're not too sure about having a stranger touching you. Or your girlfriend 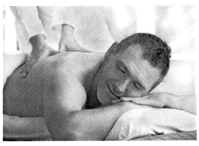 wants you to at least *try* a pedicure – but you get embarrassed at the thought of anyone inspecting your toenails too closely. That's perfectly understandable, but you might be missing out on something important.

The essential, underlying message of this book is about using spa as a tool for taking charge of your personal health and wellness and reducing stress in the process. Looking and feeling good are the bonus side effects. Not just for women, but for men, too. And speaking of looking good, you're probably among the growing number of men who know that a well-groomed appearance is a major plus in today's highly competitive business world.

All this could be true, you say, but I'm still not completely convinced.

First of all, you're not alone. Statistically, men make up around 20% of day and medical spa clientele and around 30+% of resort spas', so there are obviously many men out there who either don't know about the benefits of Spa-going or still see it as a "girlie" thing. Yet over 50% of spas, especially in hotels and resorts, have added a selection of men's treatments to their menus and are going to be happy to see you when you walk in the door.

So what's holding you back? Oh right. A spa is full of women. Don't worry, once you understand what to expect, it's a piece of cake! And who said that a little pampering is for women only?

Let's get started. What we won't do is repeat the information in Chapter 3 "Getting the Most Out of Your Spa Experience." The mechanics of going to a spa are the same for men and women. However, there are still a few things you can look for from a guy's point of view to make sure that you find the right spa experience.

We'll also take a brief look at what makes a man's skin different from a woman's, what you can do for your skin at home and then examine the more popular men's treatments.

 ## Finding the Right Spa

More likely than not, the woman in your life will have some excellent input and be able to steer you in the right direction, but if you want to do your own research, here are some things to look for in addition to the advice in Chapter 2.

Go online, take a look at a few spa treatment menus and look for their men's sections, often listed as "services." Compare them, decide which spa most appeals to you and then give it a call to see how male-oriented it really is.

In some cases, spas have added "treatments for men" to their menus that are simply their regular treatments with a more manly name. A good yardstick is to ask whether they use products "specifically formulated for men's skin" and have men's skin care products for sale, since the products they use in their treatments and those that they offer for sale go hand in hand.

And it might be that you'd be more comfortable in a hotel or resort spa, since men tend to make up a smaller percentage of clientele in day spas. The most important thing is that you take that first step.

Get Down to Spa Basics

Now that you've decided to take that first step, let's look at what spas do to make a guy like you feel comfortable in addition to the treatments for men most commonly found in today's spas.

Spas that are truly serious about their male clientele feature:

- Neutral colours and furnishings that appeal to both men and women,
- Seating large enough for male frames,
- Well-appointed men's change rooms,
- Easy to understand messaging in their treatment menus,
- Reading material/magazines of interest to men and
- A good selection of men's skin and body care products for sale.

5 Things to Think About Before Your Treatment

1. Does the spa's robe cover you adequately?

If you're a big guy, you might want to check with them in advance, and if you have to wait in a co-ed area, please, ahem, remember to keep your legs together.

2. Do you have a big, booming voice?

Most spas are all about a quiet, serene atmosphere and keeping your voice down is greatly appreciated, especially in the areas around treatment rooms.

3. Is your cell phone permanently attached to your head?

Try, try to leave it in the change room with the rest of your belongings and turn it off before you do.

4. Can you manage a quick shower before having a massage or body treatment?

Not only will it relax you, but your therapist will appreciate your thoughtfulness.

5. Are you a little modest?

You can wear whatever makes you feel most comfortable, but for massages your best bet is to remove all your clothing. Check with your therapist and let her or him know how you feel. My guy leaves his briefs on, so it's definitely up to you.

Treatments for Men

Massage

Massage is the single most favourite men's treatment and a perfect way for you to start your spa journey. In Chapter 5, check out the 10 Steps to a Terrific Massage to find out about the process and make sure you're getting the most out of it. You don't have to be a professional athlete to appreciate all the benefits a good massage provides. Whether you opt for a sports massage, a relaxation massage or any other of the massages listed on a spa's menu, you'll feel great afterwards. Why?

Massage in its many forms:

- Lowers the sensation of pain in your body,
- Increases restorative nutrient-rich blood flow to your muscles, cartilage and ligaments,
- Reduces your body's levels of the stress hormone cortisol,
- Elevates levels of dopamine and serotonin that can help alleviate depression and anxiety,
- Lowers heart rate and blood pressure and
- Strengthens your body's immune system making it more capable of fighting everything from stress-related problems to the common cold.

Face Treatments

Even though you might be sure you're already taking excellent care of your face, neck and chest, it's still a good idea to have professional skin care about four times a year as the seasons change.

Like most men, you're probably more performance and results-oriented (and less interested in the pampering aspects of a facial, except perhaps the relaxing massage). So, you'll be looking for face treatments that deep cleanse, reduce oiliness and 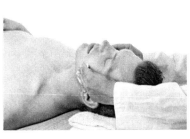 moisturize your skin, leaving it clean and fresh. There are a number of traditional spa skin care lines like Kerstin Florian, Pevonia, Elemis, Decleor and Comfort Zone that have come up with specialized products for men that are geared to do that.

Your spa therapist will examine your skin in detail and then, depending on your skin type, tailor a face treatment that addresses your particular concerns to give you the best experience possible.

The Process:

- To get the most out of your treatment, shave just before your facial unless your facial includes a barbering service.

- After a thorough cleansing of the pores, you'll receive an exfoliation or scrub that freshens your skin and gets rid of dead skin cells on the skin's surface.

- Either a steamer will be used or hot towels will be wrapped around your face to open your pores. Due to your skin being more oily than not, you will most likely need to have those pesky blackheads (if you have any) removed through extractions. Though this sounds more like mining for ore, it really is as simple as popping those little bits out of your face using nothing more than a Kleenex and your therapist's fingers. Don't worry, since your pores are already wide open at this point, you should experience only minimal discomfort.

> If you find extractions too uncomfortable, simply ask your therapist to stop. You don't have to continue. And if you have rosacea or very sensitive skin this step may be modified or omitted altogether, since heat will exacerbate your condition. Other products will be used to purify and calm your skin, instead.

- A face massage will follow to relax you and at the same time stimulate the flow of oxygen-rich blood up to the surface of the skin that helps move the toxins out of the tissues of your face, into your bloodstream and on into your kidneys for elimination. Men say that the face massage is the best part of the treatment!

- Depending on the type of face treatment you receive, there might be a masque applied to your entire face and neck that will give your skin the additional nutrients it needs to keep it healthy.

- When your therapist removes your masque and finishes up, your skin will feel fresh, clean and look great!

Back Treatment

One area of your body that often needs extra attention is your back because, no matter how hard you try, there are places there that you just can't reach. Give it the attention it deserves and discover why this treatment is another favourite for most men who enjoy going to spas.

The Process:

- Starts with a deep cleanse using specialized products.

- An exfoliation and/or scrub (see face treatments above) follows to remove any remaining dead skin cells and steamy towels are applied to open the pores.

- Impurities like blackheads will be removed if needed, but if it's too uncomfortable, ask your therapist either to stop or keep it short.

- A masque will possibly be applied to the entire back that the therapist will choose based on your skin needs.
- A lotion will be massaged into your back for a great finish.

Note that spas love to individualize their treatments, so you might find variations on the above.

 Cold Beer, Anyone?

The last couple of years have seen the use of beer, malt, yeast, hops and barley in spa treatments designed to appeal to North American men. It's actually not as gimmicky as it sounds because the vitamins and minerals in these ingredients can be truly beneficial for the hair and skin. The best news is that most spas that feature beer in their treatments serve the beverage nicely chilled *during* the treatment as well as in it.

Put Your Foot Down

As far as your feet are concerned, you no doubt are one of the millions of men for whom flip flops or sandals are your "go-to" summer footgear, so keeping those tootsies looking great makes good sense.

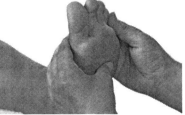

The most important consideration, however, is the health of your feet. Regular pedicures mean that conditions like toenail fungus and athlete's foot can be intercepted and dealt with by someone who knows what to look for and how to handle anything questionable before it becomes a real problem.

The Process:

- Feet are soaked to soften the skin and cuticles,
- Nails are cleaned and cuticles are pushed back,

- Cuticles are trimmed with special nippers or with a special liquid remover,
- Nails are filed and shaped,
- Any calluses on the soles of the feet and toes are removed,
- Feet and lower legs are massaged and
- Nails are buffed.

You won't always need to change into a robe and should either wear shorts or be able to roll your pants up above the knees so the therapist can do her job most effectively.

Hands Up!

If you're a guy in the business world where appearances "make the man," well-manicured hands are an absolute must. On the other hand (no pun intended), if you're a guy who makes a living with his hands, taking good care of them could provide much needed relief.

The manicure process is similar to a pedicure: soaking, cleaning, cuticle care, filing/shaping, massaging the hands and arms and buffing. Most spas, including resort spas, include a simple, stripped down, no-frills version.

Most guys just want to get these treatments over and done with in as little time as possible. Consequently, treatments for men's hands and feet tend to last from 30 to 60 minutes at the most. Some spas that offer hair care will provide a manicure while you're having a haircut and in some cases you can get a manicure while having your pedicure. If you're in a time crunch, it's a perfect way to go, so be sure to ask if it's possible.

Opt for a resort with a good spa and book a side-by-side pedicure with your wife or significant other the next time you're on vacation. Follow it up with a romantic side-by-side massage and you'll both think you've died and gone to heaven.

Make Someone Happy

Did you know that going to a spa could actually put a smile on your face? In 2005, KSL Resorts completed an interesting survey that revealed that of all men polled, 35% believed that spa going could lead to an improved sex life. However, and this is really interesting, of the guys who actually were spa goers, 60.4% reported that, in fact, spa going actually *did* improve their sex lives!

Men Are From Mars and Women From Venus

Following are some handy tips on keeping your skin healthy and looking good outside of the spa. Some of them might surprise you!

Believe it or not, your skin is different from a woman's. It's about 20-25% thicker – excluding the underlying fat. Your face has smaller oil-producing sebaceous glands, which feed into the hair follicles that are more active than women's thanks to your testosterone. This makes your skin oilier and your pores often larger, causing your skin to be more prone to breakouts and acne as a result. You also tend to sweat more and in different areas from women.

But the biggest difference? You have more facial hair and it's coarser and denser than a woman's. OK, that's no surprise, but unless you sport a beard, you're probably also shaving at least once a day, right? What may come as a surprise to you is that shaving makes your skin more sensitive than a woman's as a result. Did I say sensitive?

It's important to understand what happens to your skin when you shave. Whether using a straight-edge or electric razor, the blades regularly remove not only the hair but also bits and parts of the outer layer of the skin. In fact, shaving creates microscopic nicks, no matter how new the blade, that need to be quickly repaired to prevent bacteria from invading and causing infection. We often perceive these nicks as irritation or razor burn for which men's aftershaves and colognes were once thought to be the answer. Today, we know that the alcohol content in those products actually caused the skin to become dry and probably did more harm than good.

Not only "razor burn," but also itchy, irritating ingrown hairs are often a problem. Then there's that tight feel to your skin that you experience after washing that you might mistake for that "squeaky, clean" feeling. The only problem is that your skin could actually be dehydrated or lacking moisture and in dire need of something that will replenish it.

As a man, you need skin care products with formulations that specifically address the differences between your skin and a woman's. Whether in the drug store or spa, the good news is that you'll now find a wider variety of men's skin care lines — thanks to an increased demand for "men's care" as a result of men's growing interest in it.

Face It - Your Skin Care Routine

The old KISS rule — Keep It Simple Stupid — when it comes to taking care of skin seems to work best for most guys (the simple and not the stupid part!) and I'm guessing you're one of them.

Here's a quick and easy routine to keep your skin clear and healthy over and above shaving:

One. Cleanse with a gel or lotion that can be washed or sponged off. Every evening! Do not, and I repeat, do not use your favourite hand soap. Sure it cleans your face, but it also strips the protective outer barrier of the skin and can lead to visible signs of aging, not to mention irritation and dryness. All the men's skin care lines now offer cleansers that address your manly skin type, including dry, oily, sensitive and stressed. To help close pores after cleansing, splash cold water on your face. Rinse your face with plain water or in the shower in the mornings — a cleanser isn't necessary.

Two. Exfoliate at least once to twice a week. That means using a product that has small beads in it that remove dead skin cells and deep-cleanse the pores so that your moisturizer is more easily absorbed. There are also special cloths that will do the job. However, since this step may be more than you are ready and willing to do, having a deep-cleansing facial every couple of months is a good way to keep dead skin cells from building up.

 ## What's His Secret?

My 93-year-old father-in-law has skin that puts men 30 years younger to shame — few wrinkles and a smooth, healthy appearance. He's worked outdoors and done a lot of living, so what's the secret? Good genes or good skin care? Probably both since he has been caring for his skin faithfully his whole life with fairly simple products like Nivea and he told me, "That includes my feet!"

I peeked in his medicine cabinet and found a facial cleanser, an exfoliant and a moisturizer. He says it makes his skin feel better!

Three. Moisturize with a balm or lotion after you cleanse your face whether you shave or not. Your skin needs the active ingredients present in these lotions every bit as much as a woman's. If you can find a lotion that contains a sunscreen, so much the better. If not, apply a sunscreen after moisturizing — but don't forget it. The sun is the single biggest culprit in damaging your skin (see Chapter 8 on sunscreens). Another plus for you is that many men's care products combine ingredients that address more than one issue, recognizing that most men want to keep it simple, convenient and quick.

As far as body care is concerned, though I heartily recommend using a moisturizer after showering, I also realize that it might be asking a lot of you. At least that's what my husband tells me. So do what he does and use a moisturizing body wash rather than a harsh soap when showering. It will get you just as clean as soap without completely stripping the skin of its moisture balance.

So, do you feel a little more comfortable about going to a spa and taking care of your skin like it deserves? I really hope so!

And we've only skimmed the surface of all the things that a spa has to offer — regardless of gender. There are a number of other treatments like wraps and scrubs, sports and fitness activities, nutrition counselling, meditation and lifestyle programs, such as cooking, music and photography classes, for you to delve into and enjoy. Not all of these activities are found in all spas, but when they are available, indulge your curiosity and give them a try.

Book a spa vacation at a dude ranch or a ski resort or on a remote island for something really different. Check www.experienceispa.com, www.spafinder.com, www.leadingspasofcanada.com, www.destinationspagroup.com or www.spasofamerica.com for a good list of resort and destination spas. Better yet, google the spas in your own hometown and get going. Once you start, you'll get hooked!

Chapter 5   Ummm, Ummm Good - Massage Anyone?

Just got back from a massage.....in Mexico. Los Cabos, to be exact, a thousand miles south of Los Angeles on the Baja Peninsula and famous for its elegantly gracious, award-winning spas housed in equally beautiful hotels and resorts. Coming from British Columbia, well known for having some of the most stringent and exacting standards for registered massage therapists in the world, I was curious to see just how professional their massage therapists would be. The spa I chose was beautifully appointed, but could its therapists match in terms of expertise?

I was pleasantly surprised. My expectations were exceeded and I left feeling relaxed, fluid and centered. The tightness in my shoulders was gone and I felt two inches taller!

I've had massages in Germany, France, Switzerland, Austria, Greece, Canada, China, the USA and once on a Russian riverboat! Some were very, very good, a few were extraordinary and a very few left me feeling worse than when I started. Most, however, delivered exactly the kind of massage I was looking for (and needed at the time), leaving me feeling more fluid, relaxed, centered and balanced.

In this chapter, we'll examine the benefits of massage, look at the 10 steps to a terrific massage, when not to have one, some of the most popular massages found in spas, where to go to find a reputable massage therapist and, finally, see how massage can benefit those with cancer.

Benefits of a Good Massage

Massage has been around in nearly every culture, stretching back thousands of years. Today is no different, with men and women from all walks of life opting for the many benefits of massage on a regular basis. They book their treatments in spas, hospitals, rehab/health centres, with mobile services at home and in private massage practices.

For you, it's a terrific way to begin your spa journey and is a vital element of the health and wellness spectrum as you decide to take responsibility for your own wellbeing.

In the spa, it shouldn't come as a surprise that the treatment of choice for reducing stress and inducing relaxation continues to be a massage. And speaking of stress reduction, it remains the number one reason globally for visiting a spa.

In fact, nearly every part of the body can benefit from massage, from fingertips to the top of the head to the soles of the feet. Massage in its many forms:

- Lowers the sensation of pain in the body,
- Increases restorative nutrient-rich blood flow to muscles, cartilage and ligaments,
- Reduces the body's levels of the stress hormone cortisol,
- Elevates levels of dopamine and serotonin that can help alleviate depression and anxiety,
- Lowers heart rate and blood pressure and
- Strengthens the body's immune system making it more capable of fighting illnesses.

 What Science Says About Massage

An excellent resource for discovering how extensively the many benefits of massage have been scientifically researched over the years is the Touch Research Institute at the University of Miami School of Medicine.

Dr. Tiffany Field, director of the Institute, explains that one of the primary benefits of touch seems to stem largely from its ability to reduce levels of cortisol, a stress hormone manufactured by the adrenal glands, leading to enhanced immune function.

The many studies conducted since TRI was formally established in 1992 further support the beneficial effects of massage on everything from autism to osteoarthritis to bulimia. In nearly every study, a decrease in anxiety, pain and/or stress levels was reported.[2]

Recently, a supporting study undertaken at Cedar-Sinai Medical Center in Los Angeles concluded that even a single session of Swedish Massage Therapy produces "measurable biologic effects," notably significant decreases in cortisol in the blood and saliva and also in arginine vasopressin, a hormone that can lead to an increase in cortisol. Further, it showed an increase in the number of lymphocytes, a necessary part of the immune system. The study concluded that if these findings are replicated in further studies, it might have "implications for managing inflammatory and autoimmune conditions."[3]

In addition, there have been thousands of other studies conducted here in North America and around the world that demonstrate the benefits of massage for a wide variety of conditions (see http://www.spaevidence.com).

Scientific studies aside, what this means for you is that after a good massage you can expect to feel better and be a little healthier! And the best news is that you can specifically target "what ails you," whether it's stress, lower back pain, sitting too long hunched over a computer or a sports injury.

10 Steps to a Terrific Massage

I. Booking your massage

When booking a massage, don't hesitate to give your preference for a male or female therapist and the preferred intensity of your massage. Most therapists can give a variety of massages, but not all can perform, for example, deep tissue work. And if you're looking for some of the specialty massages, especially aromatherapy, hot stone, cranio-sacral, Lomi Lomi or Thai, you want someone who is well trained in that particular modality and knows what they're doing. Ask.

Give the spa a heads-up at this point as to your physical condition, if necessary. Are you pregnant? Do you have any allergies or any medical conditions they should be aware of? Although you will be asked to fill out a guest history form (or at least should be asked to do so) when you check into the spa, letting them know beforehand will help them book the best therapist for you.

You might also want to ask whether the facility has change rooms and/or provides robes and slippers. Some do and some don't. If they don't, you'll most probably remove your clothes in the treatment room and slip directly onto the massage table.

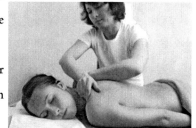

If you have any other questions or concerns, now is the time to make them known.

Massage Therapist - Male or Female?

This question has been floating around for years. It is often argued that male therapists, because of their physical strength, can give a deeper massage, while female therapists tend to listen more and massage more intuitively.

Whether you are a man or a woman, you will probably have a preference for one or the other, but if you are in a situation where your preferred gender is not available, refusing the other gender might be short changing yourself. Again, it comes down to communication: asking for medium or deep pressure or directing him or her to work on specific parts of the body.

If you can, get referrals from friends or family. The therapists' credentials are also a yardstick for the success of your massage, i.e. where they've trained, the number of hours they've trained and/or the quality of the spa and its staff in general (though not a guarantee in all cases).

2. Relax beforehand

Do yourself and the massage therapist a favour: if you haven't had a steam or refreshing swim, at least try to shower before heading into your massage. Aside from the obvious benefit for the therapist of having a clean body to massage, water is the ultimate soother and your aim is to become as relaxed as possible before your massage so that the therapist doesn't have to spend the first part of the massage loosening up your tense muscles. You'll definitely get more out of your massage if you do!

3. Check-in in good time

Arrive at least 15-20 minutes before your scheduled start. It doesn't matter whether it's a day or stay spa, it will give you time to fill out the guest history/medical form and change into your robe and slippers, remove all your jewellery and hit the bathroom one last time. Time, too, to pause, take a couple of deep breaths and clear your mind of all the day-to-day "stuff" that's whizzing around in your head.

4. Meeting your therapist

This is when you begin to consciously establish your energy rapport. Okay, so not all of us are outgoing or can talk easily with strangers, but like I say later in the chapter, establishing a personal relationship – if only for an hour – really is a two-way street. Whether male or female, they will most likely introduce themselves and ask you a few questions regarding the type of pressure you prefer, where you're from, etc. Be friendly, forthcoming and honest in turn, particularly if you have any conditions you want addressed, such as a sore lower back or tension in your shoulders.

And even though you filled out the client form, it's not a bad idea to reiterate any personal issues you might have. For instance, the vein on the inside of my left ankle going up into my lower leg has given me problems since I was 17, so I always ask my therapist to go easy around it. Or with my hypothyroidism, I don't do well with someone massaging my throat area.

It's especially important when you don't speak their language. Generally, they speak enough English to be able to introduce themselves and ask your name, but from there on in, it's all eye contact and body language!

5. On the Massage Table

As you are ushered into the treatment room, you will be asked to disrobe and get under the sheet, lying either on your stomach or on your back. The therapist most often will leave the room while you do.

OK, so now you're lying there on the massage table waiting for your therapist to re-enter the room. A few minutes pass and then a few more. Will the time be deducted from your massage, you wonder? Finally the therapist comes bustling in and the massage begins. Except that you're still wondering about the clock and not concentrating on the massage and all that energy business.

How do you get around it? When you're ushered into the room, you might tell your therapist that you only need a second to disrobe and slip under the sheet and, if *you* don't mind, ask her to stay in the room while you do (although in some places this is actually prohibited by law). Say so in a friendly way, or simply ask how long she'll be out of the room. Even if she still needs to leave you — perhaps to wash her hands, fetch more massage oil, etc. — she'll be alerted to your desire to get on with it.

As you arrange yourself on your stomach, managing to get the sheet up around you, don't forget to make sure that your face feels comfortable in the doughnut-shaped headrest and your hair is off your neck for easy access for your therapist. If the headrest is lined with a towel, there should be no folds or ridges that can cause discomfort the longer you lie on it, nor should it impede your breathing in any way. Though this might seem fairly insignificant, it can distract from your enjoyment of the massage experience.

6. Decent exposure

You may feel concerned at the thought of taking off all your clothes. Of course, you can always leave on panties or underwear (or more), but you'll find that it's a nuisance during the massage. I'm probably one of the most modest persons you can imagine, but because of the way a person is draped, I never feel that I'm being in any way improperly touched (this is pretty blunt, I know, but it bears mentioning).

 A Word About Draping

This is a technique that every massage therapist worth his or her salt in North America observes religiously. As mentioned, you'll be asked to lie on your tummy or back under a sheet. If you're like me, you're fairly modest and would prefer to remain covered, rather than lying exposed to someone else's eyes.

As the therapist massages you, each body part (whether arms or legs; your back or your front) will be individually exposed. The sheet will cover the rest, with the linen around the inside upper thigh area tucked in under the unexposed leg during the leg massage. When you turn over, he or she will hold the sheet up at eye level so that you can do so comfortably and then drop the sheet down over your body, again exposing only those areas being worked on. While lying on your back, some therapists place a small hand towel over the breasts (under the sheet) so that you remain covered while they work on your front side, especially during abdominal work.

On the road, you'll find that most international spas that have a reasonably large North American clientele are good about draping, although not everywhere.

Of course, the main reason for removing your clothes is to allow the therapist to perform the massage most effectively, but do what makes you feel most comfortable – especially you fellows who might be a little worried about your "dangling parts."

I'll never forget one of my very first massages, which happened in the 80's in Germany. I was instructed to remove all my clothes and lie face down on the massage table. I did and the male massage therapist placed a small towel over my bum. I wasn't completely comfortable but decided to just hang in there. However, he proceeded to ask me to turn over on my back and there I was, feeling like a turtle on its back (and just as helpless). The only saving grace was that he didn't seem in the least discomfited, so I kept my eyes screwed shut and made it through. As you can imagine, the only thing I remember about that massage was my embarrassment at being so totally exposed. I didn't have another massage for a long time after that!

The long and the short of it is not to do anything you're not comfortable doing. So, leave on (or off!) whatever you feel will be most comfortable and beneficial for you.

7. Starting the Massage

In every good massage I have ever received, the therapist takes a minute or two having you either breathe deeply and exhale fully for a few breaths or using some other calming/centering technique. As you do, she either pushes gently on your back as you exhale or initiates contact with you in some gentle way. Give into it and let your mind go blank, concentrating on nothing more than your breathing. Be fully in the moment and let everything else fade into oblivion...

8. Massage no-no's

No touch zones during a massage are the buttocks and legs near the genital area, the genitals themselves or the breasts for women (unless a specific breast massage). It is not unusual for the outer sides of the buttocks to be included in the upper leg massage or the upper part of the buttocks to receive attention in the lower back massage, but you shouldn't expect a "butt" massage per se, unless your glutes are tight and sore and you request it. And for you guys, your therapist reserves the right to refuse to continue if she observes a physical reaction in a certain part of your anatomy. Although this can happen during the massage as a result of increased blood flow through the torso, and will be ignored by a true professional, inappropriate behaviour as a result will not. Definitely not part of a spa massage.

9. During the Massage

Believe it or not, this one point is another major pet peeve. My personal

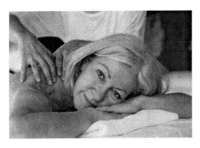

"good massage" yardstick is whether the therapist spends the same amount of time on my left leg (and arm, side of my back, feet, etc.) as he does on my right. And also whether he uses the same sequence of moves on the left as he does on the right,

regardless of the length of time I've booked. For some reason, I have an eidetic memory when it comes to the sequence of movements during a massage.

It really irritates me when he leaves out a step or two on the opposite side, giving me the impression that he's hurrying to get through. I've thought a lot about this and wonder if it has to do with whether the person is right or left handed. Maybe it's like throwing a ball – you do better with one side than you do with the other. Some day, I'm going to break down and ask!

After a few minutes, you'll be asked whether the pressure is all right. The terms "light," "medium" or "firm" are fairly subjective, so be open and tell your therapist what feels right to you. "Grin and bear it" isn't an option here.

As to the amount of time allotted for a full-body massage, is it possible to fully and effectively massage a person from head to toe — including scalp, hands and feet — in 50 minutes? Some really good therapists can and do. And if you have a massage on a regular basis, your therapist will probably focus more on one part of the body than the other at any given time, based on your needs.

But on the whole, particularly if you're not a regular spa-goer, you're best off requesting that your therapist, before she begins, focus on the specific part of your body that you know needs the attention, rather than just lying there hoping that she'll be able to read your mind.

Or even better, spend the extra cash and get a 90 minute massage so that she can devote more time to each area.

 ## Spotting Trouble Before It Begins

A couple of years ago, I had the pleasure of hearing a keynote address by Horst Rechelbacher of Intelligent Nutrients and founder of Aveda, one of the first large aromatherapy-based product lines. He was talking about all the reasons why people should visit a spa and, as an aside, he made one point very emphatically to all the spa professionals sitting there: during a massage, the therapist should always be on the lookout for suspicious looking moles or abnormalities on a person's back and body and point them out immediately. He maintained that this is one of the most valuable services the massage therapist can perform for his or her clients.

Do all massage therapists have this knowledge and training? Possibly not, but the well-trained and certified therapists should. Another good reason to regularly visit a reputable spa between your annual medical checkups, right?

10. Checking Out

Once the massage is over, your therapist will normally tell you to take your time – important since you might be a bit groggy and don't want to stumble or fall getting off the table. Also the soles of your feet might be slippery, so if you haven't been given a towel to wipe them with, take extra care.

For the sake of the guest who will follow you, though, once you feel a little more alert, please head on back to the change room or put on your clothes as quickly as you can. If your makeup or hair need touching up, and they probably will, that can be done in the bathroom or change area. Your therapist will appreciate you leaving the treatment area within 3 to 5 minutes so that she can change the linens and tidy up the room. It also gives her time to clear her energy in order to be receptive to the next guest. Before she does, your therapist will probably escort you to the reception desk unless she's running late.

You know, it's funny, but when I've had a particularly good massage, I find it almost hard to say goodbye to my therapist. A hug and a quick good-bye and I feel like a good friend is walking away from me. So I always let him or her know how much I appreciated the wonderful attention and make sure that I leave a corresponding gratuity when I settle my account at the desk.

That Special Something

As I mentioned earlier, while we often talk about the mechanics of a massage, it's probably a good idea to also address something a little more intangible that is the underlying factor that will enable you to get the very most out of your massage experience.

It's Energy.

The Chinese call it *Chi.* Traditional Chinese Medicine's Tui Na is based on keeping the body free from external and internal factors that can block the flow of *Chi* along the meridians through the body and keep you healthy. *Ki* is the Japanese equivalent and proponents of Reiki claim that it does the same –

removes blockages to the life force energy that flows through the body. In Ayurveda, it's the *Marma* points in the body that are stimulated to achieve a balance in the *Prana* or energy flow. Massages or treatments deriving from these and other healing systems are based in part on the assumption that the healing power of touch is dependent upon the exchange of energy between the person being touched and the person giving the touching.

Whether you believe this or not is up to you. I do – based on my own personal observations and experience. There are many ways in which our life force energy is kept healthy and strong and I believe that massage in its many forms is one of the most effective ways possible.

Interestingly, a study conducted by California's Institute of HeartMath[4] showed that "when people touch or are in proximity, a transference of the electromagnetic energy produced by the heart occurs." Test results also implied "that the exchange of cardiac energy described here may be influenced not only by the degree of coherence of the transmitted signal (which, in turn, can depend on the source's emotional state and intention), but also by the degree of the receiver's receptivity to the signal." In other words, when both giver and recipient are in a "mutually caring relationship" the positive effects of touch are magnified. It's important to point out that this is only a single study and that further research needs to be conducted, but most massage therapists would verify these findings from a purely personal, intuitive perspective.

Let's think about the potential amount of energy that can be transferred between you and your massage therapist during a massage treatment. To me, the difference between a truly great massage and a mediocre one depends to a large extent on the energy rapport my therapist and I are able to establish from the get-go, regardless of the length or type of massage. Consider how long the average massage lasts. During that time, you are being touched by, and as a result are exchanging energy with, another person – often someone you've never met before – with the expectation of leaving feeling relaxed, healed in some way and centered. When you think about it, it's really a bit of a gamble, isn't it?

Most of the time, since massage therapists tend to be highly intuitive, caring people, they make the effort to engage you prior to your treatment. But what happens when the therapist doesn't seem to be fully present, maybe because she has personal problems or isn't in a good space? Then it's up to me – on a strictly human level – to find a way to initiate the rapport if I want to have more than a perfunctory service. And, obviously the longer the massage, the more important it becomes to establish this rapport. It's definitely a two-way street.

As a spa director, I used to monitor my therapists, especially at the end of the day, to check their positive/negative energy levels to make sure they remained healthy both emotionally and physically. If you think that a massage is just about having your muscles kneaded, think again.

Interestingly, if the therapists were going through some sort of personal challenge or not feeling well and were unable to properly channel their guest's energy, it seemed to accumulate in them and by the end of the day they would be chalky-faced and utterly exhausted.

So pay attention to attuning yourself with your therapist to get the most out of your massage experience. It gives new meaning to the old saying "go with the flow."

What Can You Expect as a Result of Your Massage?
You should feel better than when you went in. That's the bottom line. Stress, pain and tension will be diminished as blood flow to the muscles increases and neurochemicals in the brain are altered and stimulated. You will probably feel a lot lighter in spirit than when you started, as well. And the more often you have a massage on a regular basis, the more balanced, energetic and healthy you will feel.

Remember to drink plenty of water afterwards to flush all those nasty toxins out of your system that have been released through your massage. Do expect to feel more relaxed, even possibly sleepy. If so, it's not a bad idea to sit quietly for a few minutes, either in the spa lounge or somewhere nearby, before driving a car or getting on with it.

In some cases, especially after deep tissue work, you might have experienced moments of pain or discomfort as specific areas were worked on. Don't worry, this is normal. Often, an area adjacent to the one that was addressed will seem sore, but that's just because your whole system needs a bit to get back into a balanced state. Give it some time and if you have any problems, let your service provider know.

When NOT to Massage

❀ *Varicose veins*

Deep pressure should not be applied to areas with varicose veins. Light pressure using the flat part of the fingertips and palms can be used, but deep finger pressure, cross-fiber friction, tapping and stripping movements should be avoided[5]. However, light lymphatic drainage strokes or the short movements used in a circulatory massage, always stroking toward the heart, can be beneficial.

❀ *Medical Conditions*

Massage is not recommended when you have infectious or contagious skin diseases, like dermatitis and inflammatory conditions of the skin; moderate diabetes mellitus; advanced heart or kidney disease; venous problems like deep vein thrombosis or phlebitis; highly metastatic cancer; fever and quite a number of other conditions or diseases that would ordinarily be treated by a doctor. A more complete list, provided by the College of Massage Therapists of British Columbia, is listed in the Resource Guide.

If you have any questions whatsoever about varicose veins or any of the above conditions, please check with your doctor before scheduling your massage.

12 Most Popular Types of Massage

Full-Body Massage

This 50-90 minute massage treats the entire body from the top of the head to the bottoms of the feet. It avoids the breasts, the buttocks and inside of the thighs near the genital area and the genital area itself. Generally, the face will not be fully massaged. If you have identified a specific area of concern like the back and/or shoulders, given time constraints, take into account that your therapist might not be able to spend as much time on the arms and hands or front.

And, as regards the front, while you're lying on your back, what can you expect? The neck and décolleté (the area between the base of the neck and the tops of the breasts), the muscles of the thighs, the lower legs, the feet and often the abdominal area will be addressed. If lying on your back 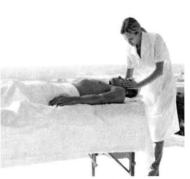 makes you feel a little vulnerable, tell your therapist who will do what she can through draping to make you feel as comfortable as possible.

Swedish Massage

This technique is the basis for a number of massages such as deep tissue, relaxation, aromatherapy and sports massage. Mainly a vegetable/fruit-based oil, such as grape seed, sunflower, almond or apricot kernel, is used that is first applied to the therapist's hands to lessen the friction of the hands moving over the skin and to allow long flowing strokes to be applied to the more superficial layers of muscles.

The strokes (known as effleurage) are stronger in the direction of the heart and lighter moving away from it. She or he may use forearms and elbows in addition to hands to stroke and/or apply pressure. During the treatment, the therapist may also use kneading, rhythmic tapping, gentle shaking or friction movements. At first the pressure is light, becomes more intense as the treatment progresses and then becomes lighter again towards the end. It should never be uncomfortable for any length of time, although if an area of the body is knotted or overly tense, it can be – and I use this word advisedly – somewhat "painful" while the therapist works the kinks out.

⭐ Please note (and I have had this happen) that if the pressure is too intense or deep, your body will tense up in response producing the opposite of relaxation. So, again, be clear with your therapist. My worst experience occurred when I was a spa-going beginner and kept thinking that the therapist would let up. Before I knew it the massage was finished and I felt like I had been worked over with a meat cleaver. Not good!

Aromatherapy Massage

The entire nervous system can be positively or negatively affected through your sense of smell (olfactory stimulation). Aromatic herbs, trees, flowers and other plants provide a wide variety of essential oils that are used in the treatment of a number of ailments or simply to induce a feeling of relaxation and reduce stress, both through inhalation and absorption directly into the skin.

A skilled aromatherapist will help you decide which oil is most effective for you, based on your health history (some oils can produce adverse reactions in certain people depending on their health problems), and will mix the essential oil with the massage oil (carrier) being used. Pressure is light to medium depending on whether it is intended for relaxation or sore muscles. The point of the massage is more about the oils being applied and allowing them to do what they are intended to do as they are absorbed into the bloodstream over the next few hours. The most frequently used essential oils in massage include rosemary, lavender, peppermint, lemon, rosehip, geranium, sandalwood, eucalyptus, grapefruit, chamomile, neroli, ylang-ylang, juniper, sage and jasmine.

Since some persons react negatively to certain essential oils, it is imperative that you smell the oils the therapist intends to use before beginning the treatment. If you don't like the smell, decline its use. Your nose knows. As I stated above, some oils should not be used in the case of specific medical conditions – so be diligent in filling out your guest history form so that your trained therapist can make the appropriate recommendations. As well, many aromatherapy oils cause photosensitivity of the skin (sensitivity to sunlight), making it more prone to sunburn, including tanning beds. Brown skins should also take especial care when using them and many essential oils are not recommended for pregnant women.

And one more tip: rather than showering after your massage, remove any excess oils from your body with a warm towel so that the oils can keep on working after the massage is over.

Manual Lymphatic Massage

Light, rhythmic massage pressure stimulates the movement of lymph fluid through the lymph system, composed of lymph nodes and channels between that remove waste, microorganisms and other foreign substances from the tissues into the bloodstream so they can eventually be eliminated. This massage can help effectively boost the immune system, reduce swelling in ankles, legs and around the eyes, and promote detoxification of the body in general. It should be performed by someone trained in the technique, so be sure to ask whether the spa has therapists with this training if you're interested. For diabetics; where clots or thromboses are suspected or for those with heart or circulatory problems, it is **not** recommended.

Sports Massage

This massage is good not only for athletes, but also for individuals with injuries, range of motion difficulties and chronic pain. The different types of sports massage either prepare muscles for a certain activity; are given after an event to restore the muscles to normal; for rehabilitation of specific injured areas or to prevent injury. The therapist will generally spend most of the time on the area in question using medium pressure similar to that used in Swedish massage.

Deep Tissue Massage

The therapist goes beyond the outer layer of surface muscles to the layer below, as well as into the connective tissue (fascia). Pressure is correspondingly more intense and suggested for those with chronic pain, engaged in heavy physical activity, range of motion difficulties, with osteoarthritis or muscle tension. It works by breaking down the adhesions that form due to injury or chronic muscle tension in muscles, tendons and ligaments. It is a specific modality and should not be confused with "deep pressure" when requesting such a treatment.

There are certain conditions for which deep tissue work is not recommended: for those with open sores or skin diseases; osteoporosis; tendency towards blood clots or with heart disease; immediately after surgery or chemotherapy; or on parts of the body that have suffered even mild trauma, like bruising. If there are any questions in your mind, check with your doctor.

Hot Stone Massage

Traditionally, basalt stones have been used in this therapeutic massage, although snowflake obsidian (harder and less porous than basalt) and even jade are being used. This massage is generally more expensive and usually 70-90 minutes long.

All those photos of stones along a bare back are somewhat misleading. A hot stone should never be placed directly on skin unless it is moving in the therapist's hand. A properly trained therapist will use special draping with a double sheet to allow hot stones to be wrapped before being placed in the client's hands or on their feet. Once they have cooled from hot to warm, they can be placed directly on the skin. Some hot stone massages also include chilled marble stones used in conjunction with the heated stones.

In the traditional hot stone treatment, the stones are used by the therapist in two ways: first to transfer heat to the body by laying warm stones under the client (for example, under each shoulder when prone) or on top of you (for example, along the spine starting with the sacral stone, graduating to smaller stones at the base of the cranium). You're given an egg-sized stone to hold in each hand; similar sized stones are cradled in the foot arch. Smaller stones are often placed between your fingers and toes.

While these strategically placed stones deliver concentrated heat in key areas of the body, the therapist massages you with heated stones held in the palm of his or her hand. The stones transfer heat to your body surprisingly quickly. As they cool down, they are replaced with fresh stones, ensuring that continuous heat is used throughout the treatment. The weight and density of the stones allows the therapist to easily modify the pressure, and many therapists feel that providing stone therapy is easier on their (the therapists') hands and joints. These stones are used to deliver both deep and superficial massage over the course of the treatment.

 Recent Email From a Dear Friend

"All I can say is that I am sooo mad about the hot stone massage I had two months ago. It was terrible and now I know why. The stones were only used at the end and they were simply placed along my spine. Afterwards, all I could think as I settled the bill was, 'That's it?' It just didn't seem any different than my other massages and now I know why."

Lava Shell Massage

This is used primarily in relaxation massages where light pressure is indicated, with Tiger Clam shells that come from the Philippines. Heat in the shells is generated by a chemical reaction of the oils and seawater that are mixed with dried sea kelp, minerals and algae that are put into the shells. The heat can be fairly intense at first, but the shells cool quickly as they are moved, managing to hold their heat for up to two hours. The highly polished shells are cupped in the therapist's palm and moved over the body using the Swedish massage technique.

Do NOT have a heat related massage if:

- You're pregnant;
- You have a neurological condition that results in altered sensation or temperature perception;
- You're taking any prescription medications, which alter the perception of temperature or
- Your skin reacts to the Hot Stones or shells by becoming red and hot.

Lomi Lomi Massage

Performed with continuous, flowing strokes, using the forearms as well as the hands, this massage art originated in Polynesia (in particular, Hawaii). It is a good example of energy work, since a primary focus is to remove energy blockages within the muscles and joints to promote healing and wellness. It can vary from light to vigorous, depending upon the needs of the client, and comes from a place of love and nurturing in the practitioner.

Shiatsu

Primarily a finger pressure massage that can also use palms, arms and feet, it is given on a mat on the floor. No oils are used and you are dressed in comfortable, loose fitting clothing such as shorts and a T-shirt. By applying pressure along the meridian points of the body, blockages of chi (the body's energy) are eliminated to optimize its flow. It is preceded by an assessment to determine what specific concerns you may have and provides a wide range of benefits from improved flexibility to increased blood circulation, increased mental clarity and general wellbeing.

Thai Massage

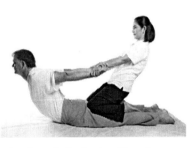

Thai is also performed on the floor, with you dressed in comfortable clothing, and is more energizing and rigorous than conventional massage. The therapist stretches your body in a series of yoga-like moves using hands, knees and legs and nearly the whole body. She also uses compression and shiatsu-like pressure point techniques during the hour to two hours of the massage to relieve muscle and joint tension and, like shiatsu, to increase the flow of energy throughout the body. It's probably not the best massage for a spa newbie due to the close contact between you and your therapist, but its benefits, especially in terms of improved joint mobility and energy, make it a tempting massage to try if you find a spa that offers it.

Reflexology

This treatment lasts from a half hour to an hour and is performed primarily on the feet, though it can also be done on the hands and ears. It's a combination of small massage strokes and pressure point manipulation applied to specific points on the tops and bottoms of the feet and toes that correspond to specific organs and parts of the body. Like other massages, this treatment balances the various systems of the body, relieves tension and improves circulation.

 Oh, Those Tootsies

A friend of mine, a lovely, sophisticated and well-known wedding photographer, was a regular at our spa. She spent a lot of time on her feet and when she came into the spa asking for something other than a Swedish massage, I suggested a reflexology treatment, explaining in detail what it was all about.

I was standing at the desk talking with one of our receptionists a little later when I saw this same lovely lady crawling out to the reception desk on her hands and knees, much to the amusement of everyone present.

"Good heavens," I said, "what are you doing down there?" She replied, "I never knew how important these feet of mine are. How can I possibly walk on them??!" Needless to say, we all had a good chuckle.

Indian Head Massage

This ancient technique, also known as Champissage, covers the neck and shoulders as well as the head. The neck and shoulders are first deeply massaged to remove any muscle tension and then the head and scalp. The therapist claws lightly over the scalp, as if shampooing the hair, to increase circulation and improve the blood supply. Next, she performs a facial massage, and finally gently rubs the forehead, moving from the centre down each side of the face to the temple. Besides feeling wonderful, it removes tension from the shoulders and neck, releases sinus pressure and relieves stress that can ultimately lead to headaches.

Of course, there are a number of massages that I haven't covered that you might be curious about: couples massages, pregnancy and some of the more esoteric massage treatments. For instance, there are a number that are based on "energy work" such as Reiki, Esalen, Tui Na, Amma, cranio-sacral and others that might appeal to you. If you're interested in the variety of massages performed today, take a look at a fairly comprehensive list and their descriptions at www.ncbtmb.org/consumers_glossary.php. And if you see something on the spa menu that piques your interest, don't miss the opportunity to be enlightened and ask!

Who's Qualified

This is an area that deserves some scrutiny. It is your right to ask where the spa's massage therapists and body workers have been trained and if they have the proper certification depending on the type of massage you're looking for. If you need a massage due to an injury or for more specialized work as opposed to a relaxation massage, you might want to google the National Certification Board for Therapeutic Massage and Bodywork (certifies massage therapists in 35 U.S. states) or the American Massage Therapists Association for qualified practitioners and massage schools in your area. In Canada, refer to the Massage Therapy Alliance of Canada at www.massage.ca with chapters in seven provinces and one territory. For other massage types such as relaxation, acupressure, shiatzu, etc., visit the website of the Natural Health Practitioners of Canada for listings in your area.

Some states and provinces require 500-1000 hours of training and in British Columbia, the most rigorous, 3000 hours. The difference between those therapists without rigorous training and those that have had it is the degree to which they can be considered "simply" relaxation therapists or whether they can actually be considered part of the medical health care system.

Even in states or jurisdictions without licensing, there are different requirements and standards that may apply. Until there is regulation at the federal level in both the U.S. and Canada, there will continue to be a discrepancy from one state or province to the next. So, again, if you have concerns, contact the associations above, as well as the International Spa Association and Spa Industry Association of Canada to find reputable spas with qualified practitioners in your area.

Internationally, your best bet when traveling is to google "Massage Therapist Association of (Country)" and see which have licensing and which don't. Sweden and Italy, for example do not, while Germany and New Zealand do. At www.globalspasummit.org you'll find a list of associations from around the world dedicated to advancing the professionalism of their therapists. So, be sure to do your homework and try not to leave it up to chance.

A Word About Spa, Massage and Cancer

It sounds so brutal, but the fact is that around 50% of men and a little more than a third of women will be diagnosed with cancer at some point in their lives, a cataclysmic and dire event that can have profound physical and psychological repercussions for the patient. At a different level, these repercussions extend to the person's family and loved ones, as they too deal with the disease. And even when the disease has been cured, the "cure" itself – whether radiation, chemotherapy or both – can have physical consequences for years thereafter.

It's no wonder that many people affected by cancer seek the solace and diversion that a visit to the spa can provide. The power of touch can help them feel more whole and renewed in body and spirit, better able to cope with the stresses imposed by the disease.

Yet at the same time, there are a few points that need to be considered on the part of both the therapist and the guest, if these goals are to be realized.

The disease and treatment can cause skin to become more fragile; the immune system less able to deal with infection; and energy levels to become generally lower, with the result that some spa therapies, including massage, place undue stress on the body. And since the lymphatic system is already hard at work flushing the powerful toxins of chemo and radiation from the body, additional stress from heat, deep pressure or detoxifying body treatments can lead to unpleasant and sometimes dangerous outcomes like lymphedema. As a rule of thumb, chemotherapy takes a year, and surgery and radiation six months, from which to recover.

According to Gayle MacDonald, author of *Medicine Hands: Massage Therapy for People with Cancer and Massage for the Hospital Patient and Medically Frail Client*, there are many reasons for spa therapists to be less demanding in their treatment of even former oncology patients. Here are a few of them:

- Easy bruising,
- Fatigue,

- Immunosuppression,
- Loss of bone density (can be due to steroids, the disease process, metastatic spread to bones, radiation therapy or certain chemotherapies),
- Pain medications,
- Peripheral neuropathy in the hands or feet and
- Risk of lymphedema.

In addition, vital organs such as heart, lungs and liver may still be healing or in some cases may be permanently damaged from the toxicity of chemotherapy or due to scarring by radiation. Consequently, a too-heavy massage could trigger the symptoms that were experienced during chemotherapy. As well, the results of nodal involvement can last for many, many years and if these areas are massaged too vigorously, it can lead to lymphedema in the arm that could be permanent.

But this doesn't mean that massage or other spa treatments need to be avoided altogether. You just need to take a few precautions. Please note that the suggestions below are solely to help you, the spa and your spa therapist be more aware of your condition – not to replace the professional medical advice of your physician:

❋ *Information is crucial.*
This is especially important if you are not a regular guest at the spa. Even though explaining might make you feel uncomfortable, the therapist must know if you have or have had the disease and its location, particularly if you have had lymph nodes removed from or radiated in the neck, axilla or groin or have any condition that makes the bones more fragile. Your fears that the therapist might refuse to treat you – for whatever reason – are greatly outweighed by the risks to your health.

❀ *Be aware that not every spa therapist understands the impact on the body during cancer treatment.*

A detoxifying wrap or lymphatic massage can unduly overload the lymphatic system, as discussed above. You need to be very clear in stating the parameters for your spa treatment and not agree to something that you feel or know would be detrimental to you. A good therapist will appreciate the information and shouldn't react negatively.

❀ *Seek less demanding treatments.*

Let your massage therapist know that you prefer lighter pressure during the massage, like a gentle Swedish or aromatherapy massage, and to avoid the areas that have been affected by chemo or radiation. Try a Vichy shower or have a facial, and avoid detoxifying herbal, clay or mud wraps or an exfoliation with coarse products such as salt, sea sand, cornmeal, pumice, bamboo and ground nuts. The more frail a person is, the more necessary this is to observe and please don't put undue pressure on your therapist by demanding a treatment that she or he knows could have a negative outcome.

❀ *Make sure good hygiene and sterilization practices are observed by the spa.*

If you choose a manicure or pedicure, either as an alternative or in addition to your massage, be sure that anything used is either disposable – in the case of files and buffers – or has been sterilized.

❀ *Try not to pack too many treatments or activities into a single day.*

In order to avoid overloading your lymphatic system, especially if you are not used to the activities, try to remain aware of your limitations, if any. Pay attention to your energy levels and get plenty of rest, including between treatments.

As noted above, even though it is very much up to you to take responsibility for yourself, it is still very crucial that your physician be consulted before visiting the spa. It's also a good idea to check with the spa to see whether their therapists have had experience with oncology patients. But once there, even when you may feel at your lowest, the physical, emotional and spiritual benefits can be significant.

In closing, massage therapy, in all its guises, is a sure bet for your continuing health and wellness and thousands of practitioners worldwide are ready, willing and able to provide these beneficial treatments for you.

So, massage, anyone?

Chapter 6   Love the Skin You're In

Flip through the pages of your favourite magazine and you'll find page after page of gorgeous women — and men — of every shape and colour with silken, glowing skin showing on every visible square inch of their bodies! OK, so those models have probably been airbrushed, but still...then you look in the mirror at your oh-so-familiar face and body and what do you see? Are you satisfied or could you possibly be doing more to keep your own skin just as luminous and radiant?

In order to understand why regular spa treatments and a good home care regimen are so necessary to the health of your skin, it's important to first understand the skin itself. We'll look at how the skin functions, the different skin types, what's in a moisturizer, basic skin care tips, ethnic skin and teen skin. It's a lot of territory to cover, I know, and perhaps "a blinding flash of the obvious," but still worthwhile reviewing.

How the Skin Works or What I Learned in Fifth Grade ... and Forgot

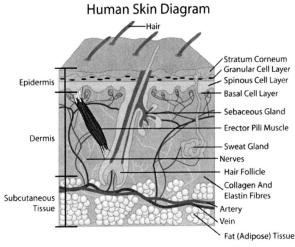

The skin is made up of the Epidermis, the Dermis and the Subcutaneous Layer, varying in thickness from 0.05 mm in your eyelids to 1.5 mm in your palms and the soles of your feet. If you are an average adult, you have around six square feet of skin weighing about 18% of your body weight.

The Skinny on the Epidermis

The epidermis, on average only 1/1000th of an inch thick, consists of four layers with different functions. The biological and chemical processes that occur in this layer are far too complex to describe here; suffice it to say that when all is said and done, the epidermis has the power to keep all the bad, environmental "stuff" out while protecting all the good "stuff" in the layers below – for me a miraculous, highly underestimated, part of the body, indeed.

For our purposes, let's concentrate on two: the stratum corneum and the basal cell layer.

The Stratum Corneum and Your Lipid Barrier

The Stratum Corneum is the outermost layer of the epidermis that consists at the outside of flattened, overlapping dead skin cells. Within this layer, often referred to as the "bricks and mortar" of the skin, the corneocytes (the bricks) are held together by lipids (the mortar) that are found in the spaces between these cells, forming the intercellular matrix, which also contains 15-20% water. It is often referred to as the lipid barrier, responsible for the barrier function of the skin that protects it from the loss of moisture and penetration by foreign substances. If it is compromised, it can result in dry, scaly and cracked skin, dermatitis, acne, eczema, congested skin and can even weaken the skin's immune system.

Water loss in the lipid barrier occurs, in part, due to external factors such as low humidity and exposure to cold and wind. Other factors that remove the natural moisture factors (NMF) of the skin include detergents, excessive use of soap and water, over exfoliation and irritating chemicals and solvents. And as paradoxical as it sounds, over exposure to water actually results in moisture loss.

As the skin becomes drier, the natural sloughing of dead skin cells is reduced causing scaly, less pliable skin.

The Basal Cell Layer
This is the bottom layer of the epidermis and responsible for producing the cells of the outer layer. These cells break loose from the basement membrane of the basal layer and travel upward through the other three layers to the stratum corneum over a period of about 28 days in a continuous process. As noted above, once in the stratum corneum, the spaces surrounding these cells are filled with lipids to form the lipid barrier. In healthy, normal skin the rate of cell production and cell loss is equal and in balance.

5 Steps to a Healthier Lipid Barrier

Age, heredity, some medications, your diet, the time of year and the state of your health will also affect your lipid barrier and, as a result, your approach to skin care needs to be *individually tailored* to its present condition.

Even though a one-size-fits-all approach isn't the answer, there are still a number of things that you can do regardless of your skin type to ensure that your lipid barrier stays as healthy as possible for as long as possible.

I. The Right Cleanser

In general, a mild cleanser or gel at night followed by a tepid water rinse is sufficient for your face. Avoid using soaps that dry it out. Some people prefer to use a cleansing lotion and remove the cleanser with a sponge or washcloth rather than rinsing with water. The main thing is to keep pores free by removing all dirt, impurities and cleansing residue from your skin before applying a moisturizer.

In the morning, rinsing your face with plain water is fine. In the shower, though, try to avoid hot steamy water directly on the face, especially if you have rosacea. I prefer to soak a cotton (not cotton blend!) pad with a mild, alcohol-free facial tonic and use it to gently cleanse my entire face and neck from the previous night's "debris" rather than use water.

Following up cleansing with a toner is also a matter of personal preference — if you do, avoid toners containing alcohol if your skin tends to be dry. Then follow up with your daily moisturizer/ SPF 30+ sunscreen.

2. Exfoliate with Care

Don't over exfoliate! Use a loofah on your body from time to time and a good, moisturizing body wash appropriate for your skin type. An exfoliating body scrub isn't such a bad idea in the summer when we're already applying oils and sunscreens that feed the lipid barrier, but in the winter, when we're contending daily with often overheated rooms, chafing clothing and cold weather, a washcloth is usually sufficient to remove dead skin cells, yet avoid further irritating or damaging the skin.

However, in the case of overly dry skin, because cells aren't turning over and shedding naturally as often as they should, it's necessary to exfoliate as often as once a day. You might want to try dry brushing, discussed later in chapter 9, to stimulate blood flow to the skin as well as slough the dead cells. If your skin still seems scaly or patchy, use a gentle exfoliant from time to time and follow up with a good moisturizer afterwards.

The same applies to your face. Don't over exfoliate or you run the risk of stripping the lipid barrier's protective oils and moisture, thereby subjecting it to the risk of infection or skin problems like skin congestion, rosacea-type inflammation and dermatitis, especially if you are overdoing glycolic acids or (mis)using do-it-yourself microdermabrasion kits and products. Furthermore, depleting the skin's moisture weakens the cells in the lower layers of the dermis and, as a consequence, the immune system of the skin.

Signs of Over-exfoliation:

- Acne, skin congestion, inflammation and irritation,
- Noticeable dryness,
- Redness,
- Increased fine lines and
- Feeling of tightness.

This isn't to say not to exfoliate. On the contrary, removing the dead skin cells that build up in the stratum corneum is a necessary part of your skin care regimen. Follow instructions for your skin type and just don't overdo it!

3. Protect Your Face and Neck

Make it a rule to moisturize your clean skin in the morning and especially at night from your hairline to your collarbone in order to give the skin a chance to repair itself. Depending on your skin type, you'll require products containing a combination of moisturizing (humectants) and softening (emollients) ingredients. The most important thing, regardless of your skin type, is that you continue to replenish the moisture and oils that your lipid barrier needs to stay healthy, from the inside out and the outside in.

And, unless you wear a ski mask when you go out, remember that you're subjecting your face to any number of environmental threats, especially in the winter when your skin is under attack from the elements, so you might want to consider amping up your moisturizer to a heavier cream – even during the day – for the most efficacious protection of your skin.

4. Sun Again!

The lipids in the lipid barrier are affected by the sun's UV rays in a process known as peroxidation that causes a breakdown in the intercellular matrix and makes it less effective in fighting the ravages of daily life. A broad-spectrum 30+SPF sunscreen applied daily is ideal – even in the winter! Or be sure to look for moisturizers and make-up that contain a sunscreen, to ensure that you do have adequate protection, even if it's only an SPF15. Some protection is better than none at all.

5. Inside Out

Feed your skin from within daily. Vitamins A, B, C and E as well as zinc and essential fatty acids all help to keep your skin healthy. And even though you've heard it a million times, six to eight glasses of water a day help keep the skin of your entire body more soft, supple and healthy.

Down to the Dermis

The dermis makes up about 90% of the skin and it's where there's a lot happening: hair follicles, the production of sebum that "oils" the skin, sweat glands, blood vessels, lymph vessels, nerve endings and the collagen and elastin fibers that hold the dermis together. This is where much of the water in the body is stored and determines how we cool our body (by sweating), how we warm our body (by increasing blood flow to the surface) and how we age (when the collagen and elastin production deteriorates).

Moisturizers, as such, do not penetrate to the dermis. Collagen, hyaluronic acid and elastin molecules are too big to move from the epidermis down into the dermis, so creams and skin care preparations containing these ingredients that make such claims are not reliable – although hyularonic acid is an effective humectant within the stratum corneum. You simply can't replace collagen and elastin topically, but you can stimulate collagen production within the dermis with certain ingredients that do penetrate more deeply such as retinols, alpha-hydroxy acids, copper peptides, and anti-oxidants like green tea, Vitamins C and E, Coenzyme Q-10 and lycopenes.

Remember that the sun or photoaging is the biggest culprit in the aging of the skin affecting not only collagen and elastin production deep down in the dermis, but also the outer lipid barrier. Your best line of defense against photoaging is protective clothing, avoiding the sun at its hottest – only "mad dogs and Englishmen go out in the noonday sun" – and ensuring that you wear sunscreen or skin care products with sunscreen in them year round.

 A Little About Eye Creams

Do you believe that your face cream will be adequate to care for the skin under and around your eyes? Not so. The skin around the eyes is much thinner than the skin of the rest of your face and your facial moisturizers simply aren't able to take care of concerns like puffiness, dark circles and those pesky broken capillaries. Specialized eye creams are designed specifically for this area, so look for ones that are appropriate for the condition of your skin.

Don't skimp and start early! Beginning in your teens and 20's will delay the aging process significantly.

Skin Types

Understanding your skin and knowing what you have to do to keep it healthy and vital is a basic part of your overall wellbeing.

In general, skin is classified as normal, dry, oily, combination or aging. As we noted above, your age, gender, ethnicity, climate, diet, medications and average sun exposure all contribute to your skin type. Different skin types react differently to the changing seasons and often need different products at different times of the year (a description of the appropriate products for different skin types follows further down under Moisturizing).

If you haven't been to an esthetician in awhile, a visit might be a good idea to see whether you're wasting money with your present skin care regimen or are still on the right track. And, of course, to keep your skin in optimal condition, regular facials at a reputable spa are highly recommended.

What's in a Moisturizer?

As the name implies, a moisturizer is meant to replenish and help retain moisture in the skin to enable the lipid barrier to do its job. In most cases, it contains active ingredients that are usually a combination of humectants and emollients/occlusives; water (65-85%); preservatives; emulsifiers and fragrances. The combination of these ingredients determines the ways in which they replenish and repair oily, dry, normal, combination and aging skin to keep it healthy. In the past five years, research has given us a better understanding of how the skin actually works, allowing the skin care industry to develop products and technologies that are more targeted to specific conditions and better improve their effectiveness.

Humectants

These ingredients serve to pull up moisture into the lipid barrier mainly from the dermis (and attract it from the air with a 70%+ humidity) that lubricates and fills in the spaces between the cells. They can be considered the cosmetic equivalent of the natural moisturizing factors (NMF) present in the skin. These include glycerol (the most effective), isopropyl palmitate, hylauronic acid, aloe vera, urea, alpha hydroxy acids and lactic acids amongst a long list of others. Desirable for all skin types, humectants help keep the skin plump and moist.

Emollients and Occlusives

Ingredients such as almond oil, jojoba oil, lanolin, squalene, shea butter, mineral oil, tocopherol, wheat germ, silicones and beeswax act to prevent the loss of surface moisture from the skin. They should be applied to damp skin and are recommended for dry skin along with humectants, as both these ingredients help the skin retain moisture. They are often greasy and some of these ingredients may cause clogging of pores, especially in oily and acned skin, so be sure to look for the term "non-comedogenic" on products containing them.

Other Active ingredients

Antioxidants such as vitamins A, C and E help neutralize those nasty free radicals that age the skin. Fruit acids and essential oils containing antioxidants have beneficial properties that calm and condition the skin or boost the skin's natural immunity. There are a number of other ingredients including peptides, animal proteins and vegetable proteins that are added to the natural, cosmeceutical, anti-aging, organic, botanical and "other" products that we use to keep our skin healthy.

Emulsifiers

Common emulsifiers include sodium lauryl sulfate, sodium laureth sulfate, cetyl alcohol and lecithin that allow water and oils to remain in a suspended form in lotions and creams. These sulfates can cause problems for sensitive, including acned, skin in which case a sulphate-free shampoo is recommended.

Preservatives

A sticky subject, this. Preservatives make up 0.1 to 1% of the total ingredients in a product and are necessary to prevent bacteria and/or fungus from forming, prolong its shelf life and keep it safe to use. Nevertheless, many of the preservatives, especially parabens, that have been used in skin care preparations for years, have come into question as being harmful. The arguments for and against are compelling, so if you do have concerns, read the labels, do your own research and come to your own conclusions. Having said that, the FDA (as of 2007) concluded, after extensive evaluation of available information and studies, that methylparaben, ethylparaben, propylparaben and butylparaben are safe as used in cosmetics and that "at the present time there is no reason for consumers to be concerned about the use of cosmetics containing parabens." The FDA further advised that it will continue to evaluate data in this area and keep the public advised.

Reading the Label

Here are a few other terms you should keep in mind when choosing your moisturizer:

* *Dermatologically Tested*

Means nothing! The term can be used even if only one dermatologist "tested" the product and doesn't ensure that it has undergone rigorous testing.

* *Non-comedogenic*

For those with oily skin and prone to breakouts, very important! It means that the product will not clog pores and lead to blackheads (comedones) and other skin disruptions.

* *Hypoallergenic*

Provides no guarantee and is only less likely to cause an allergic reaction. In general, it indicates that there are fewer fragrances and other chemicals or ingredients that are potential allergens.

* *Anti-aging*

Generally contains sunscreen or sunblock that retards photoaging and/or alpha/hydroxic acids, plus other active ingredients like ceramides, lipids, proteins and fatty acids that are supposed to repair or counteract the effects of sun and the general aging process.

* *Expiration Date*

The amount of time a product can safely be used under normal conditions and use. Please note that storing in a warm, moist area can reduce its shelf life.

More Tips to Keep Skin Healthy

Towels and washcloths

Make sure that they're changed frequently, especially washcloths. Bacteria and germs are transferred back to the skin after multiple uses if your washcloth isn't rinsed well and allowed to air-dry in between usage (bacteria do not thrive in a dry environment). And go easy with your towel when drying off after a bath or shower – too much friction can actually damage your skin. So pat your skin, rather than rub it, until slightly damp and moisturize immediately (see below).

In the shower

Do we really need a daily shower? If you're into heavy physical activity that causes sweating, of course you'll want to shower it off, but just keep in mind that water and many soaps, especially anti-bacterial soaps, strip the oils from your skin (hot water is one of the worst culprits). If you do shower daily, read the following carefully.

If you suffer from rosacea (see the explanation at the end of this chapter), try to avoid contact with hot water directly on your face as this tends to produce further redness; and if you have skin problems like acne or overly dry skin, keep the length of your showers as short as possible and the water temperature warm, not steamy hot, as well.

As for soaps, you really only need to use soaps to attack those areas that need it – private parts and underarms. Other than that, according to a number of sources, plain water is perfectly adequate. If that isn't enough for you, look for body washes containing emollients that actually add nourishment to the skin.

Long soaks in a hot, hot bath might be the ultimate in relaxation, but do so infrequently and instead of adding oil to your bath water, apply an oil-based product (not your bath oil!) directly to your skin before stepping into the bath. It will help keep the hot water from leaching oils and moisture from your skin.

Moisturizing

After you shower, make sure that your skin is still slightly damp and *immediately* apply your favourite moisturizer to lock in the moisture and hydrate your skin. If your skin is dry to normal, look for humectant-rich products such as creams and heavier lotions. If you have oily skin, you should consider gels, serums and lighter lotions, including avocado, almond and mineral oils (you still can use creams as long as they are labeled non-comedogenic so they don't clog pores and worsen acned skin). If your skin is "sensitive" (which can be due to both internal and external factors), you should avoid products with perfumes and dyes and use products that contain soothing ingredients such as aloe, allantoin and calendula. This applies to sunscreens as well. The time of year also plays a role and you might need a heavier cream or lotion in the winter than you do in the summer.

A good reference that explains your skin from just about every angle in easy to understand, yet comprehensive, terms is *Simple Skin Beauty: Every Woman's Guide to a Lifetime of Healthy, Gorgeous Skin* by Dr. Ellen Marmur and Gina Way.

A handy online reference with lots of useful information is www.dove.com or www.dove.ca, though not as in-depth as Dr. Marmur's book.

And for a good list of the ingredients found in cosmetics and skin care products, see Paula Begoun's Cosmetic Cop.

 Let's Get Scientific

It goes without saying that the texture, elasticity and luminosity of the skin change the older you get, regardless of your background.

Aging of the skin is the result of two main elements: intrinsic aging, which is to a great extent determined by your genetics and extrinsic aging which is caused by environmental exposure, primarily UV light. In areas of the body exposed to the sun, these two processes occur at the same time.

Basically, in intrinsic aging, the process affects cellular metabolism throughout the entire body, not just the skin, resulting in a diminished capacity of the cells to multiply and resulting in their attrition.

Extrinsic aging, more commonly termed photoaging, also involves changes in cellular metabolism, leading to visible changes in the epidermis and dermis and comes from exposure to the sun, even a few minutes a day. Other external factors that prematurely age your skin are stress, environmental pollution and poor nutritional choices, further exacerbated by repetitive facial expressions, gravity, sleeping positions and smoking.[6]

It follows that aging can be at least moderately controlled through lifestyle choices. The daily use of sunscreen is a must. In addition, recent studies show that aging can also be controlled through diet and exercise.[7]

More and more studies are emerging that suggest specific dietary supplements like white tea,[8] resveratrol[9] and curcumin[10] that seem to inhibit the process which allows a cell to change into a cancer cell (telomenses) could also have anti-aging effects at the cellular level.

Ethnic Skin

Without getting too technical, it's important to talk about skin of colour (and for the sake of simplicity, we'll include all non-Caucasian/fair skin under the heading of brown skin). Brown skin derives from Asian, Indian, African, Latin, Middle Eastern or North/South American origins and can vary from ebony to dark chocolate to light tan. It can be more yellow if you're Asian or reddish brown if Native American, with variations in colour depending upon the part of the world you come from or a particular racial mixture that results from a blending of different cultures, ie. Spanish, native Indian and African. It's a broad and varied category with many obvious differences. But there are also a great number of similarities, so let's look at them.

Black, white, yellow or brown, your skin's colour depends on the amount of melanin produced in it. Melanin acts, to a certain extent, as a natural sunscreen with the average dark skinned person having a natural SPF of around 13-15. However, brown skin can still develop cancer and is susceptible to the sun's harmful rays, so it is necessary for daily use of a sunscreen with UVA and UVB protection that reflects the sun's rays from the skin's surface (see Chapter 8 on Sunscreens). Very dark skin should use a minimum SPF 15 and the lighter your skin, the higher your SPF should be. Please note that certain medications and medical conditions may make it necessary to wear a higher SPF sunscreen as well, so be sure to ask your physician if you have any concerns.

Various factors can cause the melanin in brown skin to change – actually producing excessive melanin that can lead to hyperpigmentation and melasma (dark patches) or losing melanin in the case of vitiligo. The sun is a major culprit, but so are, as mentioned, medications including those for high blood pressure, diabetes or heart disease. Rough treatment such as scrubbing too hard with a loofah or using harsh abrasives can also stimulate your skin's melanin production. In addition, brown skin can react differently and often more severely to acne, eczema, psoriasis and other skin conditions than white skin.

On a more positive note, light skin generally ages sooner and more visibly than brown skin because brown skin doesn't wrinkle as deeply as white skin, although it still tends to loose elasticity and sag as you get older.

Ethnic Skin Care

And what to look for in skin care? In general, skin is skin – either dry, normal, oily or combination regardless of its colour. But, in many cases, your skin is a little more sensitive to certain products and you should treat it a little more gently. Moisturizers are extremely important in order to keep your skin from developing a grey or "ashy" appearance. Do avoid:

- Cleansers, toners or astringents containing alcohol, propylene glycol, fragrance or dyes,

- Products containing essential oils (concentrated oil extracts from plants),

- Moisturizers containing fragrance, lanolin, dye, alcohol or propylene glycol,
- Sunscreens containing fragrance, oil or PABA,
- Makeups containing oil,
- Alpha-hydroxy acid in high concentrations or at certain pHs and
- Detergents and fabric softeners containing fragrance, dyes, or preservatives.[11]

In other words, pay attention to labels when shopping for your skin care products! There are a number of skin care lines that have been developed especially for darker skin, but they aren't necessarily all good. Most reputable spa skin care lines have products that are suitable for you – it just means reading labels, checking with a spa esthetician and doing your homework.

Please note that, if not administered properly, many treatments found in medical spas, such as Botox®, peels, IPL (Intense Pulsed Light), laser therapy and collagen treatments, can cause changes in pigmentation or result in skin damage. Since medical spas often keep before and after photos, ask to see some examples of treatments they have provided for their clients with brown skin to ensure that their protocols are suitable for you. At the very least, they should be able to tell you how often they provide these treatments in a given period of time.

One thing remains a constant, however, regardless of the colour of your skin: proper home care, including the daily use of a good sunscreen, and regular visits to your favourite skin care professional.

Teenage Skin

Welcome to the wonderful world of teenage skin! Hormones, changes in your metabolism, stress and the environment seem to have changed your skin overnight from the clear, beautiful skin of childhood into a battle for supremacy over the zit monster. Maybe it's not that bad, but for most of you teens the changes are often frustrating and challenging.

 ## Kids and Apricot Scrubs

My granddaughters — sisters fifteen and seventeen at the time — had been having trouble with their skin with tiny red bumps on their foreheads as well as "zits" on cheeks and chin. They had "tried everything." On an overnight visit, we finally had the time to look at what they were using to cleanse and moisturize their skin. Turns out that they were using a dime store apricot scrub almost nightly and using no moisturizers at all. Their skin was in fact badly dehydrated, which paradoxically triggered excessive oil production.

They didn't realize that they were stripping their natural lipid barrier (see above) and removing the natural oils and moisture that keep the skin soft and supple, drying it out and making it susceptible to infection — those nasty little red and white bumps. They couldn't get over the fact that "dry," badly dehydrated skin could break out as badly as much maligned oily skin.

They both started a regimen of gentle cleansing morning and night, a weekly gentle, non-abrasive scrub and a daily moisturizer suitable for young skin. Both girls' skin improved dramatically.

What is most important to understand is that your skin reacts differently from older skin types and has different needs. The good news is that there are steps you can take to help keep your skin reasonably clear and healthy or at least minimize the breakouts.

Acne and Breakouts

Teen acne is mainly the result of hormonal changes in both young men and women, causing an over-production of sebum (oils that lubricate the skin and keep it supple) in the pores that tapers off in the late teens and early twenties.

Blackheads and white heads (called comedones) and cysts, pustules or nodules happen within the pores as a result of a whole string of physiological events. A good description of this process can be found at www.acneguide.ca.

A recent study[12] conducted in Melbourne, Australia points to a connection between a teen's insulin levels and acne. Though more research is indicated, veggies, whole grains, grain-fed beef, seafood, fruits, low-fat dairy and foods rich in Omega-3 fats seem to keep the production of sugar in the blood lower and your skin clearer. It just means giving up breads, fried foods, junk foods and so many of the foods lot of teens love. It's a choice only you can make.

But there are other factors that contribute:

- Some oil-based cosmetics, especially cosmetics shared between friends or that are old and possibly contaminated with bacteria, including applicators, sponges, brushes, etc.

- Using products not labeled non-comedogenic that can block the pores and lead to more breakouts.

- Hair products that are oily or greasy; hair sprays and/or greasy or damp hair that comes in prolonged contact with the face, neck and back.

- Over-cleansing the face and stripping its moisture and natural oils, especially with abrasive exfoliants or scrubs that compromise the protective lipid barrier.

- Hats, helmets and sports equipment that come in prolonged contact with the body.

- Squeezing and picking of zits that damage the surrounding skin and that can spread bacteria and cause scarring.

- Detergents and especially fabric softeners in pillowcases, sheets and washcloths or linens not changed frequently enough (pillowcases at least twice a week).

- Some medications — check with your doctor as to possible side effects for the skin.

To cleanse and moisturize properly, use a facial cleanser especially formulated for acned skin, a toner that contains alpha hydroxyl acid to help it rejuvenate and make doubly sure that your moisturizer is non-comedogenic and free from irritating ingredients like perfumes.

Acne can range from bothersome to severe and is the cause of much psychological pain and suffering not only for teens, but also for adults who are conscious of the face they present to the public. So what to do about it? In cases where the acne is severe or resistant, with pustules and nodules that don't respond to over-the-counter treatments or other non-medical measures, do seek the medical attention of either your doctor or preferably a dermatologist. But if you "only" have pesky breakouts, whiteheads, blackheads and pimples primarily on the cheeks and forehead, some of the above suggestions might help.

Here's some startling news: dry skin can suffer an acne-like reaction that mimics the acne of oily skin! So, both skin types need to be handled differently. The challenge is to keep the lipid barrier balanced while treating both. As contradictory as it sounds, excessive cleansing can strip oils and moisture from the skin sending a signal to the pores to produce more oil. And some over-the-counter acne products may cause excessive drying of the skin with the same results. If it sounds complicated and challenging, it is.

There are many other suggested courses of action, as well as differing opinions on causes of acne, available in magazines, from product suppliers and on the web. But rather than second-guess your condition, please make a visit to a reputable spa your next step or in the case of severe acne, to your doctor or a dermatologist. Even if you're under a spa's minimum age, generally 14-16 years of age, your Mom should be able to explain the situation and find a spa that will see you and give you the advice you're looking for.

Experienced estheticians are able to determine whether your acne stems from dry or oily skin, whether your treatment regimen is the right one, what you can do to correct the problem and recommend seeing a physician if it's necessary. And, even if you are on a treatment regimen using benzoyl peroxide, Retin-A or glycolic acids, a regular visit for an acne facial (*with your doctor's approval!*) can help balance the skin and allow the medications to work more effectively. Check the spa's website first to see if it has a specialized acne treatment on its menu, or call and ask to make sure that it is set up to handle acned skin.

Deeply acned skin with cysts and pustules should receive attention from a good dermatologist who can administer prescription drugs and recommend suitable courses of action. Your best bet is a medical spa run by a dermatologist because he or she will have the equipment (microdermabrasion, LED, laser, fraxl, etc.) effective for your particular condition and for treating and minimizing the scarring from acne.

In some light to moderate cases, microdermabrasion can help remove some of the debris plugging the follicles and improve the efficacy of topical anti-acne treatments. By removing the skin's superficial protective layer, micro-dermabrasion aids traditional acne medications by increasing their penetration into the skin. A *medical spa professional* will help you decide. Just make sure that he or she has the appropriate training and credentials in the area of medical aesthetics.

All in all, whether you have teen or adult acne, there is hope and a course of treatment suited to you.

Rosacea

W.C. Fields, with his bulbous, "potato" nose, is probably the ultimate poster child for the effects of rosacea – a skin condition that affects millions of people worldwide. It can be anything from redness to bumps and pimples to actual visible blood vessels on the cheeks, nose, chin and forehead and can also affect the eyes.

There are four subtypes of rosacea with very scientific names (!) that describe the various conditions. The condition, or combination of conditions, characteristically appears after the age of 30 and advances from mild to moderate to severe, so it's imperative to have your skin diagnosed and treated by a skin specialist early on if you experience these symptoms.

When appropriate, treatments with lasers, intense pulsed light or other medical and surgical devices may be used to remove visible blood vessels, reduce extensive redness or correct disfigurement of the nose. Ocular rosacea may be treated with oral antibiotics and other therapies.[13]

The National Rosacea Society reports that several ingredients in skin care products can irritate rosacea-prone skin, including alcohol, witch hazel, fragrances, peppermint, eucalyptus oil, clove oil and salicylic acid. Menthol, camphor and sodium lauryl sulfate also can irritate the skin.

In terms of lifestyle adjustments, avoiding hot, spicy foods, wearing sunscreen, maintaining a gentle skin care regimen and avoiding stress (good luck!) and weather extremes can help. The booklet Coping with Rosacea put out by the National Rosacea Society is an excellent resource tool available at www.rosacea.org.

A Word of Advice

A professional esthetician can help identify the state of your skin (dry, oily, combination, etc.), many skin conditions you might have, from moderate to severe, and refer you to a medical professional if necessary. Your skin is one of your greatest assets and regularly entrusting it to a spa professional, while taking good care of it at home on a daily basis, is worth every penny and minute of your time.

So, how much do you love the skin you're in? Even if you don't love it, you hopefully understand it a little better now. Isn't it great to know that you can takes steps to keep it as beautiful and healthy as possible? You're worth it!

Chapter 7   Putting Your Best Face Forward

How does it happen? You catch a glimpse of yourself unexpectedly in the mirror as you're washing your hands and think, "Who *is* that? Where did those dark circles under my eyes and that dull skin come from?"

This time, you know another layer of makeup just isn't going to do the trick. A good night's sleep would certainly help, but you're in the middle of an important project and can't shut off your racing thoughts to get to sleep in the first place.

Or maybe that wonder cream your friend told you about is worth a try, except she's out of town and neglected to tell you the name of it before she left.

On the other hand, it might be as simple as picking up the phone and booking a facial. Great! So, you call the spa your friend raved about and a chirpy voice on the other end asks what type of facial you'd like. Huh?

How do *you* know what you should you be looking for! What is a European facial? An anti-aging facial? How do you know if your skin is normal, dry, dehydrated or losing its elasticity?

For some answers, we'll look at the steps involved in a typical spa facial, discover the top 10 facials, see why it's sometimes important to be a little cautious, take a brief glance at skin care products and finally learn who is qualified to perform one.

The Whys of a Spa Facial

One thing is for certain, and you've heard it a million times before, we can't stop the process of aging, right? But we *can* age with grace. One of the most beautiful women I've ever known had lines around her mouth and eyes, and was clearly no spring chicken, yet her skin had a luminosity and clarity that belied her age. I asked her what her secret was and she emphasized, "Regular facials and I've always taken care of my skin."

Yet I hear over and over again, "Why bother going to the expense of a spa facial? Why can't I just keep on with the same skin care regimen I've been using for years? What's really wrong with good ol' soap and water? And what can an esthetician do for me that I can't do for myself?"

I'm guessing that these same people probably floss regularly and see their dentist or dental hygienist once or twice a year. So why wouldn't they want to give the same regular attention to their skin by visiting a spa for a rejuvenating facial?

A facial reduces stress, improves skin texture, stimulates collagen production and helps remove impurities through lymph drainage. In addition, the skin is hydrated and nourished with professional products not readily available to the average consumer. In fact, a good facial produces many of the same benefits of a good massage.

In other words, a good facial helps you maintain healthy skin longer.

A spa facial may differ quite a bit from one administered in an esthetics or hair salon. The atmosphere in a reputable spa imparts a feeling of serenity, lowering your stress levels and quieting your nerves. This simple fact makes the facial more than just skin maintenance and elevates it to a relaxing hour or two with wonderful side benefits for your skin.

Be sure that when choosing a spa you take the time to evaluate its reputation and the quality of its staff. Today there are so many businesses listed under the heading of Spa that narrowing down your choice might seem difficult, but between word of mouth, the Better Business Bureau, online blogs, directories and spa websites, you should be able to do your homework with confidence (see Chapter 2).

When you speak with the spa, ask about the licensing and experience of their therapists – if they can't or won't answer satisfactorily, move on to the next spa. It's something they should be proud of!

Five Steps to the Perfect Facial

I've had everything from gold leaf and caviar to Intense Pulsed Light (IPL) and microdermabrasion applied to my face over the years, but a really good facial still comes down to a few basic steps, whether at home or in the spa: cleansing, exfoliation, toning and nourishing. In the spa, you can expect your esthetician to add the extraction of impurities from the skin, a massage and the application of specialized masques that deeply nourish in various ways.

Even though there are hundreds of variations, these basics are procedures that have been established over the years as norms within the skin care industry regardless of the type of facial, the colour of your skin or your age.

I. Before you begin

In most cases, you will change into a wrap-around, short robe called a pareau that fastens just above the breasts, leaving the arms free. You'll hop up onto a specialized bed that is partially reclined and be comfortably cocooned in a sheet and blanket or duvet leaving your upper chest (referred to as the décolleté), shoulders and head free for the treatment to follow.

Your esthetician will put a small towel or headband around your head to protect your hairline and then examine your skin under a magnifying lamp to determine its present condition, ie. dry, oily, dehydrated, etc. in order to choose the course of treatment and most suitable products for you. This is a good time to discuss any concerns you might have, such as your home skin care regimen,

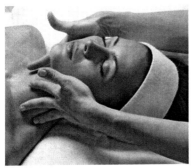

the dry patch on your cheek you're concerned about or the enlarged pores around your nose. Don't be shy – she's the professional and will be glad to answer your questions.

In turn, she may ask you questions about your eating habits, how much water you drink daily, what meds you may be taking, what type of heating you're exposed to, how much sleep you're getting and other questions that you might consider quite personal, but that will help her gather additional information to address any underlying conditions and not just the immediately observable state of your skin. Also, don't hesitate to share anything you might have done outside of your daily routine, particularly if you're on vacation. You might have a mild case of windburn from that fabulous whale-watching excursion in the morning and not even be aware of it – but you will be when she puts a hot towel on the area! If you let her know beforehand, she can cool the towel to a more comfortable temperature. Does that make sense?

It's a fact: the condition of your skin varies according to the time of year, the amount of stress you're under, your age and a number of other variables, like sun damage and your current state of health and medications you may be taking. A professional esthetician can competently assess the state of your skin and recommend the appropriate treatment. As you progress through your 20's, 30's, 40's and beyond, the actual structure of your skin also changes, requiring different treatments and products, depending upon which stage you're in. Are you able to determine all this at home by yourself?

Don't leave it up to chance!

2. The Cleansing, Exfoliation and Extractions

This very important step is the basis for the efficacy of any facial treatment. After cleansing the face with an emulsion, the skin is exfoliated with a special product that removes the dead skin cells that have accumulated on the surface of the skin, preparing the skin for all the benefits of the masques and specialized treatments that are to follow.

In some cases, your esthetician might decide that it is necessary to remove impurities, like blackheads, from your skin. She might use a steamer (a machine that delivers a fine warm mist to the face) that is used to open up the pores to make the removal of these impurities easier, although steamers seem to be disappearing from the spa landscape. Instead, she might encase your face in warm, moist towels for the same effect.

The actual extractions are done under a magnifying lamp using nothing more than the esthetician's fingers and Kleenex. Remember, your therapist has been trained to do this without damaging the skin. It's not always pleasant and be sure to tell her if the squeezing or pressing is in any way too uncomfortable or painful. You, of course, can decline the extractions in the first place, but if done on well-opened pores, it's not too awful and worth any discomfort you might experience. In any case, extractions should never be performed on cold skin – like when you're at home in front of the bathroom mirror!

Once this is completed, a light tonic, masque or cold compress is applied to the entire face to calm and ready it for the next step.

3. The Massage

So often, estheticians have a difficult time explaining the importance of a good massage. It isn't just about relaxing you or making you feel good, it's about flushing the impurities and toxins in the skin and muscles out through the lymphatic system. Massage also stimulates circulation that brings nourishment to the tissues, fed through the blood vessels from within the deeper layers.

Note: a massage may be omitted if you have had a peel because you don't want overstimulation that might lead to irritation of your skin.

The sequence in which the steps are performed may vary somewhat, but in general, the massage is given using upward and outward strokes on the cheeks; in a circular motion from outward to inward around the eyes and outward from the midline of the brow to the temples. The pressure should be firm, but not uncomfortable, in order to move the excess fluid and waste in the skin towards your lymph nodes. As in every other spa treatment, it is up to you to let your esthetician know what pressure you prefer so that she can adjust her touch.

The massage is not limited to your face and neck. The shoulders both back and front are massaged, as is the area between the upper swell of the breasts to the neck, an especially delicious and relaxing part of your facial.

Some product lines, such as Eminence Organics, have added massages for the arms and legs, performed during the masques, as part of their facial protocols (the sequence of steps employed in a treatment). Others lines may include a foot, hand or scalp massage in their facials, as well.

 Flushing What?

A well-trained esthetician understands not just the skin, but the underlying bone and muscular structure of your face and properly massages it throughout your facial to remove toxins and impurities though your lymph system. In many descriptions of facials, you'll come across the term lymph(atic) drainage and it is this process or technique to which they refer.

The lymphatic system, often overlooked and misunderstood, is located in nodes, glands, ducts and vessels throughout the body. It is key to the body's purification process, aiding the kidneys, serving the role of a filter and removing wastes. So when it is said that a facial massage helps to detoxify the skin, it means the physical act of moving and flushing the toxins into the lymph system found in the face and neck.

In general, lymphatic massage of the face and body boosts the immune system; helps ward off illness; increases vitality and health; improves the skin's appearance; reduces water retention from poor circulation or pregnancy; can help with pain and promotes the body's healing mechanism.

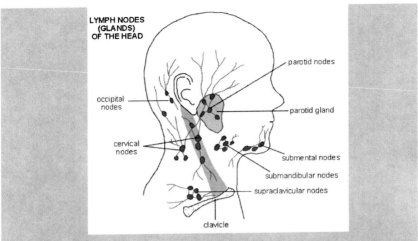

LYMPH NODES (GLANDS) OF THE HEAD

parotid nodes

occipital nodes

parotid gland

cervical nodes

submental nodes

submandibular nodes

supraclavicular nodes

clavicle

Diagram (c)EMIS 2011 as distributed at http://www.patient.co.uk used with permission.

4. The Masque

Ah – the masque! There are literally hundreds of possibilities on the market today from the very basic to the very exotic. Since your spa probably has a maximum of two or three product lines that they use in their treatments, including their own concoctions, the choices are narrowed somewhat. But even then, your therapist will have a number of products to choose from and will select a masque (or masques) most suitable for your skin *at this moment* depending on your age, the tone of your skin, its condition (dry to oily), and other factors determined by the prior analysis of your skin.

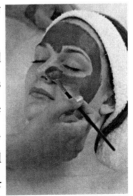

This is the actual "treatment" part of the facial and contains the most active ingredients of the products being used. In addition, concentrated serums may be used to enhance or modify the effects of the masque. They could be in the form of an add-on for a nominal fee or be included in the price of the facial. Your esthetician should tell you about any additional charges, but don't be afraid to ask if she suggests adding a particular item to avoid any nasty "surprises" at check out.

During your masque, depending on the product line being used, you might receive a hand or foot massage, a scalp massage or some other "goodie." It used to be that your esthetician would simply leave the room during the 15 minutes or so that the masque was "working," but more and more product lines are including some type of "extra" in their recommended treatments, so that you are not left alone in the room for any appreciable amount of time. In the case of aromatherapy products, check with your esthetician as to their strength, concentration and the amount being used (see aromatherapy facial below). Some aromatherapy oils cause photosensitivity of the skin (sensitivity to sunlight), making it more prone to sunburn, including with tanning beds. Brown skins should also take especial care when using essential oils and many are not recommended for pregnant women.

In some cases, a treatment line might recommend two masques, while in other very basic facials the masque may be eliminated altogether. And some spas give the massage after the masque based on the assumption that the primarily water-based masques and ampoules cannot properly penetrate skin that has been saturated with oil or oil and water products during the massage. Although the spa's menu usually indicates the steps involved in your facial, don't hesitate to ask if you're unsure.

5. The Final Step

After the masque, your face will once again be cleansed of any residual product, followed by a light toner. Finally a moisturizer will be applied and you'll be given time to allow it to be absorbed before you're finished.

Should you apply makeup at this point? One look in the mirror is enough to alarm even the most blasé of us — hair sticking every which way and skin shiny enough to light up a dark room. But unless your spa uses mineralized powders, leave the foundation in your bag, comb your hair, apply a touch of eye shadow and mascara and a bit of lipstick. You want your pores to "breathe" and the beneficial effects of the facial to continue to work in your skin.

To Talk or Not to Talk

So often I've heard, "I hate it when my therapist talks about products during my treatment." I hate it when they don't! Depending on the time of year, the skin of my face and body undergoes changes — getting much more noticeable the older I get. If a professional can't alert me to products that will remedy the situation, who will?

I also want to know exactly what she's using on my face. A good therapist or esthetician that is doing her job properly will discuss *what* and *why* she's doing what she's doing during each step of the facial. A friend of mine, and a client in our spa, once took me to task when one of our estheticians didn't, because as she said, "I don't know what I need. She's the professional and she should tell me. I can always decide not to purchase the product — that's up to *me!*"

At the end of your treatment, she will have filled out a written recommendation or she'll have put together the products that she has recommended and leave them for you at the desk. This is a service to you! Whether you purchase them or not is entirely up to you, and don't feel awkward if you don't purchase everything she has suggested.

Top 10 Must Have Facials

Anti-Aging

Designed for more mature skin, this is generally a more advanced treatment that features alpha hydroxy preparations, including glycolic or lactic acids, and beta hydroxy peels for deep exfoliation. There are strong concentrations of antioxidants in serums and masques for the face and specialized products for the area around the eyes. The skin appears firmer and fine lines may be reduced. Do allow at least a week after a glycolic acid peel before going out in the sun. These facials are best given in the fall or winter from October-April to avoid damage from strong sunlight.

Acne

Recommended for skin suffering mild inflammatory acne or with blackheads and blemishes (moderate to acute acne should be seen by a dermatologist, although there are complementary treatments that can be performed in the spa). If this could be you, and your MD agrees, look for a spa that includes it as a regular treatment and ensure that your esthetician is trained to perform one.

Deep cleansing the face of excess oils and debris that collect in the pores is the main focus with mild exfoliation and extractions performed only in the case of blackheads. A pressure point massage or lymphatic massage might be included. Because the skin is stimulated, in some cases the acne can actually seem to become worse at first, but with regular treatments and proper skin care at home, it should improve. It is very important to continue with a proper home care regimen to ensure that the skin can repair over time and to follow your esthetician and doctor's advice.

If you are using Accutane (or a related product), tell your esthetician so that she can skip the extractions and exfoliation steps and after deep cleansing, go straight to an intensely hydrating masque or application. Your skin thins out during Accutane use and can be easily damaged.

These facials can be especially beneficial for teen acne sufferers with the added side benefit of receiving proper skin care advice from their esthetician. Chances are both boys and girls will listen to a professional rather than to (nagging!) Mom.

Aromatherapy

The products used throughout the facial are tailored to your skin type and olfactory preference. Unless you are certain that your esthetician has received training in the use of essential oils, you might want to stick with spas using known aromatherapy brands such as Intelligent Nutrients, Comfort Zone and Aromatherapy Associates. In the hands of a skilled aromatherapist, essential oils, when dispersed in carrier oils such as coconut oil, are generally considered safe for use by persons of all skin types; however, some are not recommended for pregnant women or children and some can cause photosensitivity (such as bergamot, grapefruit, lemon, lemon balm, orange and others). As in an aromatherapy massage, your aromatherapist will help you decide which oil is most effective for you, based on your health history (some oils can produce adverse reactions in certain people depending on their health problems). If you have had reactions in the past, please make your esthetician aware of them.

Rosacea

This condition manifests itself as redness and swelling of the face and can lead to acne-type bumps, pimples and visible blood vessels. It is most important that soothing and balancing products are used to calm the irritability and blotchiness. Steamers should not be used and even some exfoliation should be avoided. The objective is to strengthen and heal dilated capillaries, reduce congestion and soothe reactivity for hypersensitive skin.

Pregnancy

Gentle facials are generally safe because your skin is very sensitive at this time. Things to avoid are aromatherapy, galvanic current (an electrical micro-current used to help tone muscles), microdermabrasion, deep extractions and chemical or glycolic peels.

Deep Cleansing

As it suggests, this facial is especially good for acne-prone skin due to the products, often with alpha and beta hydroxy acids, used to treat congestion and remove impurities rather than solely with extractions. It's followed up by a soothing masque to calm any redness and irritation. Having a facial that involves deep cleansing once in awhile keeps pores congestion-free and skin luminous.

Men's

A man's skin is thicker and tends to be oilier with larger pores than a woman's due to testosterone. Additionally, daily shaving can irritate and damage the lipid barrier and make the skin more sensitive. A deep cleansing facial that removes impurities, followed by products formulated for men that soothe and hydrate the skin is generally advised; in addition, the esthetician will be able to further recommend products based on the skin's overall condition.

Anti-oxidant

If your skin is dull or damaged by sun and the environment, then a facial using high concentrations of antioxidants in masques and serums such as Vitamins C, A and E, pumpkin, green tea, dark chocolate, berries, resveratrol and alpha lipoic acid could be the answer. There's a definite overlap with anti-aging facials since the objective is to rebuild and restore the damage done in the dermis by stimulating collagen and elastin production. The rest of the facial, however, is not as intensive as an anti-aging facial.

Oxygen

This facial is becoming increasingly popular due to the suggested benefits of oxygen applied in high concentrations directly to the skin. A machine that delivers up to 95% oxygen through a mist, in conjunction with a liquid solution that is said to aid in transferring it into the epidermis, is used to promote healing, brighten the skin and stimulate cell metabolism. Madonna swears by it! On the other hand, dermatologists will tell you that the skin cannot absorb oxygen into the dermis.

Signature

Every spa seems to have one. Depending on the product line used, as well as ingredients often found locally, the spa creates its own special facial that, hopefully, no one else has. They tend to be cleverly done and often are combined with other add-on treatments making them an "experience." They are

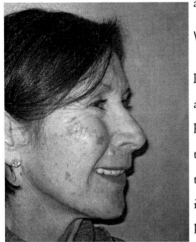

also somewhat more expensive.

When to Be a Little Cautious

There are times when you need to be a little cautious – traveling abroad and even at home. Perhaps you didn't do your homework before going to "Spa X" and then realize, at a gut level, once you walk through the spa's doors that maybe this isn't the place for you. If you decide to keep your appointment, for whatever reason, keep things simple! Have a relaxation massage instead of a more involved massage such as an aromatherapy or deep tissue massage; avoid waxing or heat related treatments or have a regular facial without the add-ons. This is not to say that this happens often or that you need to fear going to spas you're not familiar with – merely trust your instincts. And, hopefully, once you've finished this book, your instincts will be well-honed and you'll listen to that little inner voice saying "Be careful."

Why do I even bring this up? Recently, a friend of mine returned from an unforgettable trip to South Africa. After weeks of stunning, extraordinary experiences travelling throughout this vast and remarkable country, she decided to ice the proverbial cake and end her trip with a relaxing facial at a very reputable resort spa that had been recommended by a friend – and a local at that who knew the spa fairly well.

At the end of the facial, her esthetician strongly recommended waxing to remove the fine hairs of her cheeks, chin and upper lips. Normally, this isn't a problem – unless you've recently had a chemical peel or taken a product containing retinol such as Accutane. Since Sandy didn't fit either category, and even though she wasn't sure she really needed the extra service, she decided "What the heck, maybe I should."

During the treatment, she thought that maybe the wax was a little hot, but figured her esthetician knew what she was doing. However, instead of a pleasant treatment, she received painful second-degree burns to her cheeks, from chin to just beneath her eyes, just because she didn't want to offend her rather insistent, but obviously uncaring or perhaps even unskilled, therapist.

Luckily, she was able to see a dermatologist immediately after returning home. These photos show the results of one week's worth of medication and fortunately she suffered no lasting effects from the harrowing experience.

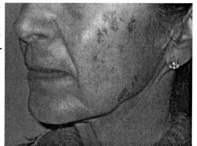

Skin Care Lines and Make-up

One thing I don't want to address in any depth is the differences between skin care lines, including makeup. Sometimes it seems like I've used or tried most of them!

There is a plethora of products each claiming to be the answer to your particular skin care concern. There are product lines for young and old skin. Cosmeceuticals containing AHA/BHA's, peptides and vitamins with advanced delivery systems and lots of other special ingredients claim anti-aging benefits. There are a number of botanical, plant-based products that proclaim themselves your skin's new best friend. And more and more organic products claiming to be free of harmful chemicals and preservatives are entering the market.

There are products for every age group, pocket book and lifestyle. In fact, on the International Spa Association's website, over 100 reputable skin care companies are listed and they're just the tip of the iceberg. And in my office I have two stacks of skin care company brochures each about three feet high!

Can you rely on the advice of your best friend or the ads you see on TV? It's pretty much trial and error if you do, and if you do, I'll bet you have a cabinet full of half-used jars and vials of skincare products. Or maybe you have found what you're looking for at your local department store on the recommendation of the skincare rep at your favourite makeup counter. I'm not suggesting that an esthetician is the only person who can recommend a suitable product line for you, but she can provide the appropriate suggestions and make it easier for you to go out and find them.

I just changed my mind. Let me go out on a limb and say that a qualified esthetician, a professional skin care specialist, is the best resource you can find (outside of a dermatologist) to analyze the condition of your skin and help you keep it healthy and vital, whether in the spa or at home.

Skin care lines, like Pevonia, Eminence Organics, Decleor, Phytomer, Murad, Yonka, Skinceuticals, Skin Authority, Sea Flora, Kerstin Florian and many, many others, provide a spa's estheticians with extensive product training so that their wide array of products can be administered most effectively in the variety of treatments the spa offers. This includes reference manuals that instruct the esthetician on the proper sequence of the products and techniques used in the treatments, providing her with the knowledge to perform your particular treatment properly and make the appropriate recommendations for home care.

So, take careful note of the condition of your skin as she describes it, while examining it under a magnifying lamp, and ask questions such as:

- *Is my skin dehydrated?*
- *Do I need a different eye cream?*
- *What can I do to reduce the size of my pores?*
- *Is there anything I can do to get rid of these little bumps under the skin?*

You get the idea! Generally, your spa will carry only two, perhaps three, major skin care lines for both professional and home care because of the variety of products required for each step of the spa's treatments and for every client's skin type. And as you might expect, the professional products used will be more intensive and powerful than their home care counterparts. At the end of your treatment, your esthetician will most probably recommend specific skin care products from one of these lines for your home regimen.

Obviously, you are under no obligation to buy the products she suggests, but if you like the way your skin looks and feels after your facial, you might want to give serious consideration to her recommendations.

Please note that the inexpensive makeup and skin care products found in drugstores and supermarkets are produced for broad consumption and tend to contain active ingredients in lesser concentrations than you'll find in product lines in spas. Though "spa" products might seem expensive, they are more targeted to your skin type, made from quality and specialized ingredients and generally require smaller amounts of product per application.

In any case, give new products enough time to actually make a difference – from 3-4 weeks – unless you experience a severe reaction. Your skin completely renews itself every 28 days as new cells push up from below causing the outer layer to constantly slough off. Your skin needs a full cycle for the ingredients to take effect. Some people make the mistake of returning products too soon thinking they aren't beneficial.

How Healthy is Your Skin Care?

Most skin care lines label the ingredients found in their products (or are required to by law). The Environmental Working Group publishes a Skin Deep: Cosmetic Safety Database where products are rated as to the ingredients thought to have potentially harmful side effects from 0-2 (low hazard) to 3-6 (moderate hazard) to 7-10 (high hazard).

Paula Begoun publishes skin care reviews and rates a wide range of skin care and makeup products. For questions about specific ingredients such as parabens, the FDA website also provides excellent information.

Who's Qualified

Throughout this chapter, I've referred to a "qualified esthetician." But what does that mean and how can you be sure that your esthetician will provide the professional skin care you deserve? I'm including this rather dry bit of information in case you would like to learn more.

Your esthetician or nail tech should have attended a state or provincially accredited beauty school or school of cosmetology (terms often used interchangeably) and received a diploma or certification from that institution. Esthetics curricula focus on anatomy and skin sciences, including how to perform facials, waxing, body wraps, make-up application and anti-aging treatments among others, along with safety and sanitation procedures. The hours required to complete a course in esthetics vary from state to state and province to province but average around 600-800 hours.

Nail care is a separate course of instruction, dealing with the health and care of the nails of hands and feet, including the application of gel and artificial nails and averages around 300 hours.

If the student has completed certification as a Cosmetologist, he or she will complete hair, esthetics, nails, makeup and possibly reflexology, with an average of 1200-1500 hours of study. After completion, many states and a few provinces require an apprenticeship of 1000 hours or more before the esthetician can apply for licensing from the state or provincial Board of Cosmetology. Nearly all states and some Canadian provinces require state or provincial licensing.

An ethical spa will ensure that its staff is licensed in their particular discipline or (where licensing is not required) that staff have completed a course of instruction in their discipline at an accredited beauty or cosmetology school. Feel free to discuss your esthetician's training and certification with the spa's manager or director, particularly if you should have any concerns.

A complete list of state-by-state licensing requirements for the U.S. can be found at www.beautyschoolsdirectory.com as well as a comprehensive overview of the requirements for cosmetology, esthetics, nail and hair. In Canada, check with your Provincial Board of Cosmetology (exact titles may vary from province to province).

A Last Word

Though a facial is one of your best bets for keeping the skin of your face and neck in good shape, it's still necessary to maintain a good skin care regimen at home between skin care treatments, get plenty of rest, eat foods high in anti-oxidants, de-stress through such things as meditation and exercise daily. Healthy skin and a healthy body go hand in hand.

And your home care regimen? Perhaps washing with a cleanser and water isn't good for your skin type and you should be using a cleansing milk or lotion, instead. Or you should avoid tonic lotions containing alcohol. Your night cream might be too rich or heavy for daytime use. The directions on your exfoliant might recommend use 2-3 times a week when you should only be using it once or twice a week. You might need a stronger anti-aging product than the one you're using.

Rather than purchase one-size-fits-all products at your supermarket or drug store, or buy into the paid programming hype on TV or even at your department store cosmetics counter, do your skin a favour and discuss these questions and concerns with a spa professional.

Just remember, your reputable spa esthetician has received hundreds of hours of training and has an in-depth understanding of all of the elements we've discussed throughout this chapter. Why don't you pick up the phone right now and book the facial you deserve? You won't regret it!

Chapter 8   Let's Look at Sunscreens

This chapter is dedicated to Alex Szekeley, a beloved and respected spa industry leader and impassioned advocate for sun protection, who succumbed at far too young an age to skin cancer (Melanoma).

The single most important thing you can do for your skin – from the top of your head to the tips of your toes – is to protect it from the harmful rays of the sun. It doesn't matter whether you are young or old, have fair or dark skin or are male or female.

What does this have to do with spas you're asking? Everything! When you look at the treatment menu of your favourite spa you'll see that at least half of the treatments are devoted to skin care. Look even more closely and you'll realize that most of the skincare treatments of the face and body are directly or indirectly aimed at remedying the effects of aging.

And since the sun is the single greatest culprit in the aging of the skin of face and body, sunscreen ranks right up there as a significant part of your home care regimen in between spa visits. No longer does a tan equal healthy, vital skin!

My skin is beginning to show the effects of my youth spent worshiping the sun. I now realize I didn't use enough sunscreen or stayed in the sun waaaay too long. I used to spend hours "getting a tan" – remember baby oil and iodine? And, let's face it, Coppertone back then wasn't what it is today.

In my late thirties, I did wise up, but years of tennis, sailing, golf and swimming (though only occasional sunbathing) have now resulted in not just freckles, but round, flat brown spots, as well as wrinkles that won't go away no matter how much body lotion I use. When I put on sunscreen today (no less than SPF 30) and don my hat for a round of golf, it's a bit like shutting the barn door once the horse is out. Of course, I'm trusting that it won't get worse if I do.

The reality is that the following statistics and words of advice weren't available in my early years. Would I have heeded them if they had been? I'm not sure, since I had no crystal ball that would show me what my body looks like now and I really did love the sun. Don't get me wrong – I'm not a shriveled up old prune – just disappointed that I didn't take the same care of my body that I have of my face.

 Fact

Science has proven that the sun is directly responsible for producing:

- Freckles and age spots,
- Spider veins on the face,
- Rough and leathery skin,
- Fine wrinkles that disappear when stretched,
- Loose skin,
- A blotchy complexion,
- Actinic keratoses (thick wart-like, rough, reddish patches of skin)
- Skin cancer.

First, a Bit About Kids

Granted, these results of sun worship aren't always immediately apparent and don't really begin to appear until your late thirties or early forties depending upon your skin type. But the reality is that at some point they will appear and you might not like what you see.

Sun damage is cumulative, starting in childhood and continuing throughout the rest of your life. Children, especially, should be creamed, lotioned and covered whenever they're in the sun – repeatedly. And infants under six months should not be exposed to the sun if at all possible since their skin is highly susceptible to burning – in just 10 minutes to be exact. In fact, one blistering sunburn in childhood or adolescence more than doubles a person's chances of developing melanoma, the deadliest form of skin cancer, later in life[14].

Have you ever noticed a child being pushed in a stroller with the sun full on its face – eyes and face unprotected – by parents wearing hats and sunglasses? I really have to stop myself from going up to the parents and giving them a good lecture.

So, pay attention to the tips below and if you have kids, apply these tips to them, as well.

Top 13 Sunscreen Tips

1. Use a sunscreen that protects against both UVA (rays that are closely linked to deeper skin damage) and UVB (rays causing sunburn), which is also known as a "broad spectrum" sunscreen and is recommended for everyone. Use it daily, year round on all exposed body parts (especially on throat and décolleté since the skin there is thinner than other areas, including the face). Check www.skincancer.org for a list of products that have been tested and that meet their standards.

2. Sunscreen in foundation wears off/breaks down after only a couple of hours so it's best to apply extra sunscreen separately, under makeup, or even along with moisturizers that say SPF 15 or higher on the label. Sunscreen formulations include creams, lotions, sprays, gels, roll-ons and moisturizers. Find a product that meets your personal preference.

3. The assumption that a base tan will help prevent getting burned or skin cancer is simply not true. Even a deep tan only provides the equivalent of an SPF 4 sunscreen in Caucasians.

4. Darker skins DO need sunscreens!! Sunscreens with a minimum SPF 15 and higher, depending on the darkness of your skin, are an absolute must for any person of any skin colour who cares not only about aging, but other harmful effects, primarily skin cancer.[15] Use them daily.

5. Always apply sunscreen 20 minutes before you're exposed to the sun to allow your skin time to absorb the product and create a protective shield.

6. Use sunscreen generously on all exposed skin, including face, neck and hands. Apply at least a shot-glass full (about one ounce). That may seem like a lot, but most persons do not apply enough to give them the protection they think they have. And be careful with the application of sprays so that they provide the amount of protection you need.

7. Store sunscreen away from the sun and heat to prevent spoiling.

8. Reapply after vigorous exercise or swimming even if the product is labeled "water proof" or "water resistant." Some very water-resistant products can last up to 80 minutes while other water resistant products only offer 40 minutes of protection. As a rule of thumb, reapply your sunscreen to exposed areas every two hours.

9. Remember that the sun reflects off water, sand and snow, so sit on a blanket under an umbrella on the beach (wearing your SPF 30, of course) and wear a high SPF on the face when skiing or enjoying other snow and water sports.

10. Take note of expiration dates. If a bottle or tube does not have an expiration date, toss it after one year.

11. Whether it's the sun or a tanning bed, both produce UVA and UVB rays that can cause skin cancer, wrinkling and sagging of the skin, brown spots and other discolorations.

12. According to the World Health Organization, no one under the age of 18 should use a tanning bed due to the sharp increase worldwide in skin cancer cases in that age group.[16]

13. Remember your sunglasses! The lighter your eyes, the more they are at risk. Regardless of the colour of your sunglasses they should meet

"ANSI UV requirements" or "UV absorption up to 400 nm" to block
99% of UV rays in order to protect against both the UVA and UVB
rays that can damage the eyes and are considered a major factor in
cataracts, macular degeneration and cancer of the eyes.

UVA and UVB Rays
So, what do you actually know about these harmful rays emitted by our
seemingly benevolent sun? Both affect the melanin that causes the skin to brown
and become tanned, but in different ways. The UVA rays cause the melanin to
break down (oxidize), while the UVB rays actually stimulate the production of
melanin. Together, the result is the tanned look to the skin still so popular
today. But both rays produce unwanted side effects.

UVA rays
A is for Aging. These rays are present during daylight hours and are the same
strength year round. 50% can penetrate clouds and about 70% make it through
glass and even some clothing and hats. The problem is that they pass through
the epidermis and disperse in the deepest layer of the skin, the dermis, playing
havoc with the collagen and elastin production that takes place there. Although
UVA rays do not cause burning, they are actually more harmful than UVB rays
and are largely responsible for the wrinkles and other signs of aging that appear
later in life. In addition, because they also damage the keratinocytes in the basal
layer of the epidermis, they can contribute to the development of skin cancer.

Unfortunately, at one time UVA rays were not considered harmful. People
visited tanning salons and tanning beds trusting that they were tanning safely.
While UVB rays, responsible for burning the skin and turning it brown, have
been largely reduced from tanning beds (now down to about 40%), the UVA
rays are still 10 to 13 times more intense than the sun. Unfortunately, the fact
that beds don't cause a burn is widely touted by tanning salons, giving
consumers a false sense of security.

A study conducted by the International Agency for Research on Cancer in Lyon, France (the cancer arm of the World Health Organization) published in Britain's Lancet Oncology in 2009 concluded that the risk of cancer increases by 75% in persons using a tanning bed before the age of 30. And according to the Skin Cancer Foundation, "The high-pressure sunlamps used in tanning salons emit doses of UVA as much as 12 times that of the sun" and "UVA contributes to and may even initiate the development of skin cancers."[17] Staggering probability, no?

Further, Dr. Zoe D. Draelos, MD, FAAD, consulting professor at Duke University School of Medicine, Durham, N.C. stated "UVA rays cause deeper skin damage and are linked to melanoma, the most serious form of skin cancer. In fact, studies show that melanoma is increasing faster in females 15-29 years old than males in the same age group. And in females 15-29, the torso is the most common location for developing melanoma, which we suspect is due to high-risk tanning behaviours - including indoor tanning."[18]

Don't be misled by websites and other sources that claim that UVA rays are not harmful because they do not burn. When was the last time you had to take something out of a window because the sun was causing fading? Wrinkles, sagging skin and cancer are OK? I think not.

UVB Rays

B is for Burning. As UVB rays hit the outer layer of the skin, the epidermis, they cause the skin to produce melanin to protect it from further damage. However, like UVA rays, they also damage and contribute to the loss of elasticity in the skin, result in the aging of the skin and are instrumental in causing skin cancer.

It simply is not true - contrary to some assertions - that tanned skin provides adequate sun protection. In well-tanned Caucasians, the Sun Protection Factor of their skin is no higher than four and for the average black skin it's around 15. In order to achieve the degree of protection we all need – an SPF of 30 – we need to use a sunscreen that brings our SPF up to 30.

And don't think that a cloudy day is protection against these rays. Up to 40% still make it through to the earth's surface. They are at their worst from 10:00 in the morning until 4:00 in the afternoon, making sunscreen protection a must, especially during these times. Year round!

The obvious conclusions? UVA and UVB rays are the biggest culprits in aging our skin and for skin cancers, like melanoma. But these effects can be mitigated or significantly lessened by taking the precautions listed earlier on in the chapter.

How Does a Sunscreen Work?

Today's sunscreens are generally a combination of both organic and inorganic ingredients and known as broad-spectrum sunscreens. The organic ingredients absorb ultraviolet rays and keep them from penetrating the skin, while the inorganic ingredients like zinc oxide and titanium dioxide actually reflect the rays away from the skin's surface. They come in a wide variety of preparations and products and are constantly being evaluated for their efficacy. Two excellent websites for information on sunscreens are the Skin Cancer Foundation and Environmental Working Group.

As far as the SPF (Sun Protection Factor) is concerned, recent findings suggest that SPF's over 50+ don't make much of a difference, perhaps as little as 1%. And though you might think that an SPF 30 would offer twice the protection of SPF 15, that's not the case.

An SPF 15 product blocks about 93% of UVB rays, an SPF 30 product blocks 97% of rays and an SPF 45 product blocks about 98% of rays.

In general, a good rule of thumb is 30+ SPF for Caucasians and a lower SPF for non-Caucasians (depending on the darkness of your skin's colour) applied daily year round. Look for products containing zinc oxide, titanium dioxide, avobenzone and Mexoryl that specifically state "for protection against UVA/UVB rays."

In the U.S., the Food and Drug Administration recently announced that in order for a product to use the term "broad spectrum," it will have to pass their test, have an SPF of 15+ and be able to prove that the higher the SPF, the higher the amount of UVA and UVB protection it provides. The product will not be able to claim that it "blocks" the sun or that it is anything more than water resistant. It may claim to protect the skin against skin cancer, but not that it prevents it.

Always keep in mind that, in addition to sunscreen, protective clothing, staying out of the sun or in non-reflective shade from 10 a.m. to 4 p.m. and paying attention to the UV Index is your best bet. And? Remember those sunglasses!

Protective Clothing

In general, dark clothing gives greater protection than lighter shades. Dark blue and black are your best bet, followed by bright colours like red and orange; and the tighter the weave, the greater the protection. Unbleached cotton, polyesters and even thin, satiny silk can be highly effective fabrics that either reflect or absorb UV rays. Water, however, reduces the effectiveness of the protection. In other words, if you put a white t-shirt on your child before going in the water, when it gets wet, the shirt provides an Ultraviolet Protection Factor of only three!

UPF Rating

Sun protective clothing carries an Ultraviolet Protection Factor much like the SPF's in sunscreen. For instance a rating of 50 means that only 1/50th or 2% of UV rays will pass through. These fabrics have been treated with special chemical UV absorbers, known as colorless dyes. Any clothing with a 15-50+

UPF can be labeled sun protective; however, most "sun protective" clothing has a 50+ UPF.

The Skin Cancer Foundation considers a UPF rating of 30-49 to offer very good protection and 50+ to offer excellent protection. To receive their Seal of Approval, sun protective fabrics must have a minimum rating of 30. For regular clothing, they recommend adding a product called Sun Guard to the wash cycle along with your detergent that boosts sun protection in your clothes and lasts for up to 20 washings.

A Canadian company, Seasons UV, makes a 50++ line of kid's swimwear called Solar Guard that's designed to alert parents with a colour change when the UV rays hit the danger level – even on a cloudy day – because the images on the fabric are sensitive to both UVA and UVB rays. Cool.

Just remember that when fabric is stretched or pulled too tight, it becomes thinner and allows more UV penetration. The same thing is true, as noted above, when it gets wet or if it is washed or worn repeatedly.

So What Are the Alternatives?

As mentioned earlier, tanning beds simulate the sun – with both UVA and UVB rays that are harmful to the skin. Leading authorities from the American Cancer Society to the Skin Cancer Foundation to the World Health Organization recommend against their use and many localities are banning them altogether. Another no-no is tanning pills containing canthaxanthin that can cause truly dangerous side effects and that are subject to regulatory action by the FDA.[19] But there *are* other, less harmful, ways to achieve a healthy, sun-kissed look.

Airbrush Tanning

In airbrush tanning, a solution using DHA, derived from glycerin, is applied by means of either a spray booth or spray gun to the skin from head to toe and reacts with proteins in your skin to simulate a tan. DHA has long been used by the cosmetics industry in a variety of ways and is considered by the FDA as safe, suitable and non-toxic for use in cosmetics and drugs to colour the skin.

Keep in mind that in the average person millions of dead skin cells are sloughed daily with the result that within a about a month the epidermis renews itself. Since the solution only darkens the very top layer (stratum corneum) of the skin, the tan only lasts between 4 to 10 days depending on how well you prepare your skin prior to the application, follow instructions for the time immediately following and how you care for your skin during the days after the application. In other words, it does fade relatively quickly.

Airbrush Tanning Tips

- Good exfoliation is key. Exfoliate all areas to be sprayed at least on the day of your service. A non-oil based exfoliant is recommended.

- Shower, and shave in the morning before your appointment or just before if possible, especially for men.

- Do not apply any lotions, moisturizers or oils to your body after showering. If you must, then remove any makeup or moisturizers when you arrive for your service.

- Schedule any esthetic or hair services or fitness activities prior to your appointment. Sweating may cause the solution to discolour your clothing.

- Wear loose fitting clothing and sandals or flip-flops, if possible.

- And after? It takes a good four hours for the process to complete. Ideally, wait at least twelve hours (or more) before showering or bathing with any kind of soap or shower gel.

- Moisturize, moisturize, moisturize! The more you do, the longer you can expect your colour to last.

- Avoid exfoliating or using a loofah on your skin while you have the tan.

- Most importantly, continue to apply sunscreen daily, as your skin is in no way protected from UV rays.

In any case, an airbrush tanning session is preferable to one from a spray booth. A spray booth uses the same amount of spray and motion over a 30-60 second period for everybody and tends not to last as long. Do some research on reputable spas or tanning salons in your area that offer airbrush tans. There are a number of systems available, so talk to friends who have had a service or go online and check consumer reviews in your community.

Self-tanning Lotions

Many skincare companies as well as actual sun care companies like B-Bronze, Coppertone and Banana Boat offer self-tanning products. Look for products that contain DHA as they work in much the same way as the solutions used in airbrush tanning. Today's products can give you anything from a "sun-kissed glow" to a deep, dark tan. However, like airbrush tanning, since only the outer layer of the skin is affected, the tan wears off within a few days making re-application necessary. Remember that they do not contain the protective ingredients of a sunscreen, so whenever you're in the sun be sure to liberally apply your sunscreen half an hour before going out in the sun and every two hours thereafter.

Five Tips for Successful Self-tanning

- Whether face or body, shave carefully and exfoliate before the application, paying close attention to knees, elbows and any other body parts that tend to look darker as they crease and wrinkle.

- Protect your cuticles and nails with Vaseline to keep them from discolouring.

- Apply methodically, first on the legs from the knees down to the tops of feet and toes, then on the thighs from front to back. Then apply to your torso and finally to your arms and shoulders. Unless you are a contortionist, find someone you absolutely trust (!) to apply the product to your back.

- Make sure to apply evenly and to pay attention to your palms and fingers. Rub them frequently with a washcloth to keep them from staining.

- Wait at least 10 minutes before putting on your clothes (staining!) and try to avoid excessive exercise for several hours after, as sweat can cause streaking.

There are also bronzers that wash off, cream tans, bronzing gels, tinted body lotions and tan enhancers. And then there are body shimmers and bronzing powders. In other words, once you get the hang of it, there's no excuse to seek the sun to get your summer bronze.

Has this helped? As I said at the beginning of this chapter, I wish I had known then what I know now. If you don't use a sunscreen daily, find one you like and start. And when you do, make sure that you're using it properly. When you hit "advanced adulthood," you won't be sorry!

Chapter 9   The Body Beautiful

It's the only one we've got! And, oh my gosh, the things we do to it. Day in and day out, this wonderful mystery we inhabit breathes, eliminates, smiles, walks, talks and just keeps plugging away even when we don't exercise, eat right or get enough sleep. Not to mention the stress we put it through!

Are you taking care of yours the way you know you should? Your annual physical, twice yearly dental check-ups and walking to work are fine, but when was the last time you gave it the benefit of a massage or a relaxing body treatment at the spa?

Remember, this isn't a "How-to Spa at Home" book. There are plenty of those to be found in bookstores or online. No, there comes a time when everyone needs the power of healing touch that is part of the many professional treatments you find at a spa. In fact, this just might be the perfect time for you to book a body treatment and take the time to de-stress and find *your* center.

In this chapter, we'll look at the many uses of water in the spa, best known as hydrotherapy, and then examine body treatments like scrubs and wraps, how they are performed and what they can do for you. Plus, we'll take a brief gander at cellulite and see what you can do about it.

Water, Water Everywhere

Water is the essence of life. It covers a little over 70% of the earth's surface and makes up about 70% of an adult's body, depending on age and lifestyle. Mother Earth can't live without it and neither can we.

From earliest times, the waters of hot springs, mineral springs and even the ocean itself have soothed and revitalized the body, mind and spirit of countless individuals in need of their healing powers. Baths and bathing in these restorative waters were integral to cultures on every continent and have remained so up to the present day. Are we any different? Where would we be without our daily shower or occasional long, candlelit soak in a tub full of soothing bath salts?

The Romans called it Salude Per Aqua or health through water and many believe that the acronym of this phrase is the origin of the word spa. Others believe the term spa originated in the centuries-old town of Spa, Belgium, famous for its mineral spring waters. Regardless, for millennia water has been considered central to the "spa" experience.

Today, there still are purists who maintain that a spa must in some way incorporate water into its programming – a view consistent with Spa's origins – and a good many do (25% of day spas and nearly 50% of U.S. resort/hotel spas include hydrotherapy in their programming).[20]

Hydro...What?

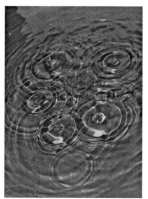

Basically, hydrotherapy is the use of water in its different forms – steam, ice and plain liquid – to relieve pain, to ease or treat a variety of maladies and to relax or reinvigorate the body. Its effectiveness has been scientifically studied and it is regaining acceptance amongst the medical community, especially for knee, hip and joint therapy (see www.spaevidence.com).

The International Spa Association offers this description of hydrotherapy treatments:

"...the generic term for water therapies using jets, underwater massage and mineral baths e.g. Balneotherapy, Iodine-Grine Therapy, Kneipp Treatments, Scotch Hose, Swiss Shower, Thalassotherapy, and others. It also can mean a whirlpool bath, hot Roman pool, hot tub, Jacuzzi, cold plunge and mineral bath. These treatments use physical water properties, such as temperature and pressure, for therapeutic purposes, to stimulate blood circulation, dispel toxins and treat certain diseases." For the sake of clarity, let's include Vichy Showers in this category, as well.

Reading through the above ISPA definition, there are a number of pretty interesting treatments. Does the Scotch hose require a kilted attendant? And what the heck is an Iodine-Grine therapy?? Since these are probably treatments that you'll ease into as you become a diehard spa-goer, I'm going to skip describing them here, but in case you're curious, I'll list a few reputable sources for further information on them in the Resource Guide at the end of the book.

So let's start with *Balneotherapy* (balneum=bath), a broad category that includes all mineral waters used in baths as well as the muds, peats and salts that are added to them for therapeutic purposes. It can also refer to plain hot and cold water treatments – just a fancier way of describing them. Balneotherapy is often considered interchangeable with hydrotherapy and it is, insofar as it pertains to baths, but hydrotherapy is actually more far-reaching in the variety of non-bathing modalities it covers.

Then there's Thalassotherapy that involves the use of seawater and marine muds, salts and kelps for their therapeutic value. When sea salts or other marine products are added to regular water, the treatment is often referred to as a thalassotherapy treatment, as well.

With regard to internal hydrotherapies like colon cleansing or irrigation, I hesitate to recommend them because of the many contraindications involved. If you are considering having such a treatment, please check with your physician before starting.

You've noted, I'm sure, how often the term therapeutic appears regarding water's beneficial aspects. Waters that are enriched with minerals, such as soda, magnesium, boron, sulphur and sodium or that come from the sea, along with the additives described above, are acknowledged for the treatment of everything from osteoarthritis to skin disorders to stress and many other conditions and ailments.

That's why if you have the opportunity to book a hydrotherapy bath at a spa, be sure to try it. Ask for a description of a particular treatment's benefits in order to find the bath most suitable for you and then relax and let your therapist and the waters work their magic.

In those spas that are fortunate to be located near the sea or at a hot springs, you will almost always find pools and tubs dedicated to the waters of that region. They can be wildly glamorous or totally simple and I urge you to be sure to take advantage of them where you find them and even go out of your way to track them down.

Okay, you say, but why would I pay good money for a bath, be it ever so special, when I can have a perfectly beautiful soak at home? Well, as we all know, it's often not what something is, but how it's provided that makes the difference. It's the professional equipment and product ingredients; the mineral properties of the water; the temperature and pressure of the water that your spa therapist employs and the yummy application of oils or moisturizers afterwards that take a simple bath to new heights. They don't just throw you into a bath, hand you a towel afterwards and send you on your merry way!

Hydrotherapy Modalities

So that you become a little more familiar with the concept of hydrotherapy, let's stick to an overview of the more basic hydrotherapy modalities you can expect at a typical North American spa.

Hydrotherapy Tub

What it is:

It can range from a simple soaker tub to a tub with over 150 air or water jets divided into zones that can be digitally controlled depending on the body areas needing attention. It usually has a separate hose for underwater massage that enables the therapist to target specific points on the body and many tubs even feature underwater coloured lights that provide salutary psychological and physiological effects on the body in a method known as chromotherapy. It can handle muds, salts, essential oils and seaweeds and most have a separate cycle for sanitizing the tub between guests.

How it works:
Whether you wear a bathing suit, bikini or other cover up is up to you and your level of modesty, but if muds, algaes or oils are added for a particular treatment, a bathing suit could be ruined. Since your therapist has probably seen just about every body type possible and only cares about providing the best possible treatment for you, it might be a good decision to leave modesty aside. Once in the tub, and comfortably situated, the jets will be programmed to concentrate on the part of your body or the particular physical condition you want to deal with, and the therapist might or might not augment the action of the jets with an underwater massage using the hose. The therapeutic effect of the water will then depend on its temperature, depth and mineral or product content.

What it does:
Circulation is improved, in turn helping eliminate toxins from the body; joint flexibility is also improved and pain and sore, tight muscles are eased. The body absorbs some of the trace elements from the various additives, which can help your skin and internal organs to heal.

Vichy Shower

What it is:
The shower is given on a cushioned wet table (treatment table with a channel around the table's perimeter leading to a drain) with shower heads arranged along a bar overhead that spray your body with water – sort of like taking a shower except that you're lying down. Coupled with a massage, it's pure heaven.

How it works:
The water temperature and/or pressure of the spray are controlled by your

therapist. It can be a stand-alone treatment, but is most often used in conjunction with body treatments to remove muds, seaweeds and other products. The spray can be very stimulating and is thought good for the treatment of cellulite. It's a pretty straightforward procedure, though if you have a problem with getting your hair wet, check beforehand to see whether the spa provides shower caps. If not, bring your own.

What it does:
Much like a hydrotherapy bath, the stimulation of the water helps increase your circulation and remove toxins from your blood stream through the lymphatic system. It will leave you feeling relaxed and less stressed.

Kneipp Therapy

What it is:
The procedures established by Sebastian Kneipp, a Bavarian priest in the late 19th century, include hydrotherapy, herbalism, diet and exercise. As a complete system, it is not as prevalent in North America as it is in Europe, particularly Germany and Austria, but aspects of Kneipp therapy are often incorporated into other hydrotherapy treatments found on this continent.

How it works:
The hydrotherapy part consists of the alternate use of hot and cold water in: *washings* using a cloth often saturated with a herbs; *wraps* that envelop the body with hot or cold cloths; *affusions* using a stream of either neutral or high pressure water applied to specific areas; *full or partial baths,* usually with herbal additives, and *water treading* in a body of water at a depth below the knee.

What it does:
Kneipp showed that alternating hot and cold water has a beneficial effect on the circulatory and the sympathetic nervous systems, as well as boosting the immune system. It can help stabilize blood pressure, increase joint mobility, relieve pain and lead to a general sense of wellbeing.

Water Circuit

A water circuit consists of alternating hot and cold therapies including saunas, steam rooms and hot, warm and cold plunge pools.

How it works:

Perhaps a specific example would be helpful. One of the most interesting circuits I've found is the Pacific Mist Hydropath at the Kingfisher Oceanside Resort and Spa on Vancouver Island in British Columbia. It takes about an hour to complete and starts with a warming massage rinse provided by a Swiss shower which comes at you from all angles followed by a mineral massage pool. Then you sit under a series of waterfalls of various volumes and intensities that massage your shoulders and scalp. You proceed to a steam cave where your body is infused with aromatic steam, after which a reinvigorating glacial waterfall brings you back to your senses.

Once you're ready, you proceed to the river walk with its warm and cool water that use the Kneipp effect to stimulate circulation through the lower legs and then on into the sea mineral soak for a relaxing float. You finish off with a mud and kelp experience in the tidal bath that draws toxins from the body while nourishing it and then, after rinsing off, relax in the lounge overlooking the sea.

What it does:

Relaxation, detoxification and stimulation are all rolled into one as a result of each of the separate waterfalls and pools with their alternating heat (causing the blood vessels to expand) and cold (causing the blood vessels to constrict).

Nordic Spas

A variation of the water circuit described above and a trend that began in Quebec, Canada is the Nordic Spa or Spa Nordique. At these mainly rustic year-round spas, a variety of hot and cold plunge pools and steam rooms combine to refresh and revive even the most stressed-out city slicker. Many offer massage treatments, are couples-oriented and located amidst spectacular nature settings.

Hydrotherapy Contraindications

Hydrotherapy may not be for everyone. If you have heart disease, are pregnant, have diabetes, abnormal blood pressure, thyroid problems, cancer or anemia please check with your physician to see whether your condition or your medications could cause an adverse reaction. And other drugs or alcohol just before therapeutic bathing are a big no-no.

Even if you have received permission from your physician to have thermal, mineral or seawater baths and treatments, be sure to alert your therapist to your condition so that if you should have a reaction, he or she can deal with it appropriately or recommend another treatment similar in effectiveness and enjoyment.

 Water As a Transformative Ritual

From One and Only Palmilla (an ESPA spa in Los Cabos, Baja, Mexico)

"A Personal Aquatic Body Therapy session. Beginning with a traditional Mexican foot and body cleansing ritual, it's a gentle form of body therapy performed in warm water. It combines elements of massage, joint mobilization, shiatsu, muscle stretching and dance. Relax even further as your therapist performs a full body massage with deeply conditioning therapeutic ESPA oils. Swimsuit required."

From Cocoon to Butterfly

Oh, where to start? The number of wraps available at spas worldwide boggles the mind while exciting the imagination. There is hardly a spa worth its salt that doesn't feature at least a couple of inventive body wraps on its menu and some spas sport such a wide selection that it's difficult to choose.

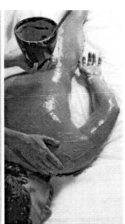

On your travels, you'll find that in their Signature Treatments – including facials, scrubs and wraps – many spas feature herbs, plants and other elements found locally. Some of these are incredibly exotic, luring us into a sensory appreciation of the spa's surrounding environment. Wraps, especially, provide the perfect medium to showcase these ingredients and are a wonderful way to creatively explore the area you're in.

10 Steps to a Perfect Body Wrap

With so many choices, perhaps it would be helpful to simply concentrate on how a typical wrap is delivered and what you can expect to do when you book this particularly wonderful treatment:

I. **Learn which wrap is the right one for you**

Just like facial products, products for the body lead to different results depending upon their ingredients. Your skin type, amount of cellulite and external factors like time of year and exposure to sun and wind will help determine which type of wrap is right for you. Nearly every spa explains the benefits of each treatment, eg. soothes dry, flaky skin; deeply relaxes through aromatherapy; invigorates the body and senses, etc. Be clear with the booking agent or your therapist as to your needs and desires and she can ensure that you receive the right one. And don't worry, just because you pre-booked a particular body treatment doesn't mean you can't change your mind once you're in the spa – providing it can be given using the same equipment and in the same time frame.

2. **Vichy or not**

   Check whether the spa has a Vichy shower that allows the therapist to completely rinse the body of all residual product. Some don't, but do provide showers where it is up to you to wash the product off, while other spas remove the product with towels. In a reputable spa, whichever method is used, there should be no "leftovers" in your bits and parts.

3. **Prepare before you go**

   As with a massage, it's a nice idea to present your therapist with a freshly cleaned and prepped body. Before having your body wrap, you might want to lightly exfoliate your body either with a loofah or light scrub with a washcloth in your shower, even though most wraps will be started with either a dry brush or wet scrub exfoliation. If it isn't clearly stated in the treatment menu, check when you book your treatment. If having a scrub, don't shave the same day to prevent irritating your skin.

4. **Consider your hair**

   Whether you are given a shower cap or not (check with the spa and bring your own, if necessary), your hair will more than likely wind up looking like you just got out of bed. Schedule your hair appointment for after a body treatment. This also goes for same-day pedicures and manicures to avoid accidental scuffing of your pristine polish.

5. **What to wear**

   Basically nothing! Before your therapist starts exfoliating and applying the product to your body, she will put a hand towel over your breasts and one over your genital area (or you might be given a disposable panty or brief) to preserve your modesty.

6. **Brush and scrub**

Now that you're capped and draped, probably lying on a mylar or thin plastic sheet that will later be – you guessed it – wrapped around you, your therapist will start with an exfoliation to remove the accumulated dead skin cells. My favourite, and one I do at home, is dry brushing. Starting at your feet with a brush made of relatively stiff bristles, your exposed skin is lightly brushed, always in the direction of the heart to stimulate your lymph system and blood flow. It begins the process of detoxification (which simply means removing any impurities and toxic substances through the bloodstream, into the kidneys and out the urinary tract, but can also include sweating). Or you might receive an exfoliating scrub that can be done with a variety of ingredients including oatmeal, salts, sugars, honey, apricot, grape/wine related, a number of plant-based oils or other products containing AHA's before your wrap. The scrub might or might not be removed before moving on to the wrap, depending on the interaction of the ingredients.

7. **The wrap**

As mentioned, wraps come in a variety of different guises and there are literally hundreds of ingredients that can be combined to nourish, detoxify and stimulate the skin of the body. Following are only a very few of those most often used:

- For hydration: many oils like avocado, rose hip, geranium, ginger, lemongrass, chocolate and shea butter are used,
- For relaxation: lavender, aloe, chamomile and lemon balm are favourites,

- For detoxification of the tissues: moor mud, Dead Sea muds and marine algaes are applied, as well as herbs like eucalyptus, rosemary and ginger and

- For improved elasticity of the skin: caffeine, ginkgo biloba, paprika, Vitamins A, C and E and green tea extract are often used and are also thought to help wage the cellulite war.

8. Wrapping it up

Now comes the cocooning part. The sheet is wrapped around you with your arms at your sides. Or you might have herbal infused cloths or sheets wrapped around specific parts of the body. Next comes a (heated) blanket placed over you to increase the effectiveness of the herbs, muds and other ingredients as they do their job and you then proceed to bake on low heat for 20-50 minutes. If you're a little claustrophobic or tend to get antsy – not to mention the need to scratch the tickle that always seems to happen on the end of your nose when you can't reach it – ask the therapist to stay with you or at least check on you frequently (although many spas today require that their therapists stay in the room with the guest). Your therapist may provide a scalp, facial or foot massage during this part of the treatment.

9. Taking it off

Depending on the facility, you're taken out of your cocoon and the wrap proper is removed under the Vichy shower. This is one of my "moments of truth" for any spa because there's nothing worse for me, as my skin is exposed to the air, than feeling chilled because the room is cool or drafty (and what might seem warm to the therapist who's moving around could seem quite cool to you). It seems like a small thing, but it can make a pleasant experience a little less so.

10. Finishing up

Once you're dried off, a moisturizer is applied in what most often becomes a mini-massage. And like post-massage, be cautious when sitting up and getting off the table. Be sure there's a bath mat when you step off and that your slippers are handy so that your slippery feet don't cause a slip or a tumble.

And you're done!

When NOT to Wrap

Did I mention claustrophobia? Right. Also, please alert your therapist if you have shellfish allergies or thyroid problems that could cause a reaction to marine products and let her know if you have high blood pressure and/or are taking any heart medications. Once again, please remember that alcohol and any form of body treatment just don't mix.

If you are claustrophobic, why not ask for a body mask instead? Muds, herbal pastes or gels are applied to the body (wrapping is not involved) and you then might spend time in a sauna, steam room or other well-heated area to achieve much the same effects as a wrap.

A Bit About Cellulite

There are literally dozens (hundreds?) of creams and lotions claiming to be effective in the treatment of cellulite. In addition to specialized body wraps, there are a number of mechanical treatments like:

- *Mesotherapy* where very small doses of different medications are injected into the affected areas to burn fat and shrink fat cells;

- *Endermologie*, an FDA approved therapy for cellulite reduction (but not removal), that is a combination of vacuum and mechanical massage to reduce the appearance of cellulite – according to the manufacturer for up to a year;

- *Laser treatments* like Thermage that do much the same thing and

- *Ionithermie*, in which clay, herbals and different algaes are applied to the affected areas to break down the fat and improve circulation, with the subsequent use of a device that employs both galvanic and faradic currents (don't ask!) that further cause these ingredients to penetrate deeper into the tissues and work their magic.

Depending on your source, these treatments are: very, somewhat, very little or not at all effective. Considering that around 90% of women over the age of 35 have cellulite on some part of their bodies you would think that there would be at least one treatment, lotion or potion that would be the answer to all our problems, and yes, I believe that I invented cellulite – starting in my 20's!

What's the answer? Yup….diet, exercise, plenty of water and a healthy lifestyle actively pursued on a daily basis and maybe one or the other of those wonder cures just might work!

Whether you have cellulite or not, regardless of the time of year, a body wrap is one of the most enjoyable treatments you'll find in a spa. And because of all the healthful benefits that water and wraps provide, you just might find yourself reaching into the medicine cabinet a little less often.

Chapter 10 Nail Those Nails for a Perfect 10

Oh, Those Tootsies

Look at any spa's treatment menu and you'll find pedicures ranging from the very simple to the often unusual or extravagant. You can have your legs, feet and nails massaged, buffed, clipped, dipped in wax, wrapped and painted in treatments taking from 30 minutes to two hours, depending upon the treatment you choose, the condition of your feet and nails and how much you want to spend.

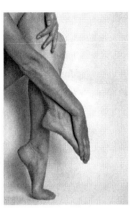

The question is whether you really need to have someone else perform this seemingly simple task rather than doing it yourself. As far as I'm concerned the answer is a resounding yes!

Most of us just aren't limber enough to get close enough to our toes to do a really *good job* of taking care of them. We also don't always have the knowledge to recognize nail problems when we see them, particularly as we get older, and once problems with our feet or nails arise no matter how old we are, they need to be addressed appropriately.

Regular pedicures can help ensure that you enjoy good foot health throughout your life and well into old age. What you do to your feet otherwise (like wearing flip flops, ballet shoes, ultra high heels or ill fitting shoes or things that negatively affect the structure of the feet) is entirely up to you.

5 Big Steps to Good Looking Feet

Whether you have chosen a spa pedicure treatment with all the bells and whistles or a 30 minute Express Pedicure, the following steps will make sure that your pedicure experience is stellar.

I. **Check out the spa**

How did you hear about the spa (or, in the case of so many manicures and pedicures, the "salon spa")? Choosing a reputable spa isn't just a catch phrase mouthed by "spa experts," it's an absolute must for all the hygienic reasons discussed below. If the spa seems less than scrupulously clean, turn around and keep looking. And when you find the one you think can do the job, check for the spa's and/or therapists' licensing where applicable. Asking is perfectly okay.

2. **Wear appropriate clothing**

You'll most probably have some sort of leg massage reaching as far up as the knee, and since not every spa provides a robe for this service, your pants should be loose enough to roll up above the knee. Also, bring flip flops or open toed shoes − even in winter − to wear afterwards or at least bring enough time for the freshly applied polish to set so that you don't ruin it (except for the UV dried polishes described later).

3. **Don't Shave the Same Day**

As a matter of fact, give it two days without shaving before your pedicure. Why? Even though you can't see them, tiny nicks are caused on your legs by your razor making it easy for bacteria to find entry into your body. It's a simple enough precaution to take.

4. **BYOI**

That is Bring Your Own Instruments. When I visit a new spa or while traveling, I always have a manicure/pedicure set with me (tucked away in my purse), including scissors, nipper, 4-way file and clipper just in case I think the therapist might be reusing the file or that the instruments aren't properly disinfected. Even if I were a little hesitant to get up and walk out, I would not hesitate to ask her to use my own tools.

5. **Give Your Nails a Rest**

Though it's nice to look down and see beautifully painted toenails smiling back at you, it's also a good idea to give those nails some time off from polish once in awhile and a chance to breathe. Since our toes are usually covered by winter footwear for at least part of the year, it's easy enough to do.

If you have any open sores or "wounds" on your feet, legs or toes, postpone your spa visit until the area in question is healed – again for your own safety. In the case of conditions like ingrown toenails, please see a podiatrist or your physician since this is out of the scope-of-practice of most nail technicians. Be sure to alert your therapist to any other concerns you might have about your feet, as well.

So, What Is the Difference Between a Spa Pedicure and a ... Pedicure?

Most spa menus list at least one regular pedicure plus their – tada – "spa" pedicure, so which should you choose? This is a question I'm asked all the time and because a spa pedicure generally costs a little more than a regular pedicure, it's natural to want to make sure that it's worth it.

The basic pedicure process is quite straightforward:

- Soaking the feet to soften the skin and cuticles,
- Cleaning the nails and pushing back the cuticle,
- Trimming the cuticles with special nippers or using a liquid cuticle remover,
- Filing and shaping the nails,

- Removing any calluses on the soles of the feet and toes,

- Massaging the feet and lower legs and

- Buffing and/or applying polish to the nails

A spa pedicure includes the same steps as a regular pedicure, but may also include:

- A specialty scrub that exfoliates and sloughs the dead skin on the feet and lower legs,

- A paraffin wax treatment to soften the feet,

- Possibly a wrap to the lower legs that helps detoxify or improve circulation and

- A longer massage and/or a variety of different massages.

As with facials and body treatments, spas draw on a wide variety of hydrating and invigorating ingredients, like lavender, thyme, menthol, allantoin and sea salts, combining them with the additional steps listed above to make a true spa pedicure more of a wellness experience than a maintenance procedure. Pedicures have always been a mainstay for all types of spas, but with spas bridging the gap between self-care and and wellness, we will see the evolution of dedicated foot care spas with "medi-pedis" and attending podiatrists similar to Canyon Ranch's "Healthy Feet" program.

A Word of Caution

In the past couple of years, there have been alarming accounts of the dangers of spa/salon nail treatments – Dr. Oz even devoted a TV show to the subject.

The biggest problem lies with the sanitation and disinfection procedures (not) carried out by some spas on a day-to-day basis. It is imperative that your spa therapist rigorously carries out the steps below to prevent the spread of infection through bacteria and fungus, including:

- Thoroughly cleaning any footbaths used for soaking the feet, including bowls and the jetted baths in throne chairs, with a hospital grade disinfectant between clients.

- Disinfection of all implements used during the pedicure and proper storage and handling thereafter.

- Single use of disposable nail files, buffers, cuticle sticks and other disposable tools.

- Preferably wearing disposable gloves, or at the very least washing her hands with an anti-bacterial soap before and after the pedicure.

- Putting paraffin wax into a plastic bag and then placing your feet in the bag rather than having you dip them directly into the hot paraffin.

This negative press, coupled with blogging on the subject, has had an impact on many people who are now worried about contracting an infection as a result of a spa pedicure. But if your spa is observing the practices outlined above, you should have nothing to worry about … other than how much to tip your therapist for the relaxing treatment!

If, however, you walk into any "spa" where the premises are less than clean or where instruments are not cleaned between treatments or reused, head for the nearest exit.

To protect the public's safety, many U.S. states have passed legislation regarding pedicure safety and most state Barbering and Cosmetology Boards have guidelines and regulations to which you can refer. The same holds true for Canada. But one of the biggest problems everywhere seems to be enforcing the regulations already in effect. So, "consumer beware" and stay alert and informed to protect your own best interests and health.

Diabetes and Pedicures

Diabetes is on the rise in both the United States and Canada. The physical consequences of this insidious disease are serious and those with diabetes are at a higher risk for infection in their feet than the average person. It is imperative that diabetics are very careful in ensuring that the above steps are meticulously observed.

If You Have Diabetes

Ask your physician if you are eligible for a pedicure, because diabetes can cause poor circulation to the lower extremities, making the skin rather more fragile. Cuts or nicks to the feet could easily lead to infection, so you'll want to avoid having your cuticles trimmed with nippers or, worse, your heels scraped with a callus razor that actually cuts the dead skin away (now banned in most U.S. states and Canadian provinces). Your best bet is to have no sharp instruments near your feet at all (nails can be filed).

If your therapist uses a callus file or rasp, just be sure that it isn't applied too forcefully and that only the dead skin is actually being removed. In fact, the whole pedicure process should be performed very gently.

It is advisable to let the spa know that you have diabetes in advance, even when your doctor gives the green light – if they can't handle you, they should let you know and you can look elsewhere. Just please, please don't look the other way if you suspect that the spa's practices are less than sanitary. You are putting your own health very much at risk.

Raise Those hands

Along with our eyes, our hands help express our thoughts, ideas and emotions. Consider how often you notice a person's hands when they're talking. For most of us, ragged cuticles, chewed nails and poorly maintained hands seem to reflect somewhat negatively on the person sporting them – a reason why most people take reasonable care of them.

Having a manicure is a lovely treat from time to time – and for many an absolute must – but is it necessary to have one in a spa rather than a nail salon, especially when you have one every few weeks? If you consider that a spa offers more than just maintenance, it would depend upon how important the ambiance of a spa is to you.

You'll find that spas offer a variety of manicures, ranging from a 30-minute express treatment to the full 90-minute Monty; however, most stop short of the application of acrylic, gel, solar, silk or fiberglass artificial nails, leaving those particular services up to a nail salon. Unless it is a dedicated nail spa, you will most probably find that if artificial nails are offered, they will typically be gel or solar nails.

If you are weighing the pros and cons of artificial nails, you'll probably want to consider acrylic or gel – still the two most popular types. Acrylic nails tend to be harder and tougher than gels and don't break as easily, while gels tend to be a little more natural looking, are more quickly applied and aren't as smelly.

For all artificial nails, look for a nail tech that has the expertise to mimic the look of a real nail including the smile or crescent moon at the base of the nail and who can apply the polymer/monomer mixture in just the right thickness. Another thing to think about is that you'll need to have the bases "filled" every three weeks or so to keep them looking good.

If you're not in the mood for a coloured polish, you might consider the ever-popular French manicure, found on some treatment menus. A white paint or polish is applied to the tips of the fingernails, and then the rest of the nails from the base to just under the tip are given a pale pink or light beige sheer polish. This gives a sophisticated, polished look to the nails that is preferred by many as an alternative to coloured nail polish and is particularly good for short to moderately long nails.

A trend worth looking into is Shellac™ by Creative Nail Design. This product is a cross between a gel and a nail polish in that it applies thinly, cures to a complete hardness in UV light in a minute per coat and can be fairly quickly removed with acetone. The company claims that it lasts two weeks, but my pedicure still looked great after almost a month (with the exception of the growth at the nail base) and I hated to have it taken off. It's very durable, free of tuolamene, formaldehyde and DBP and hypoallergenic. Other companies including OPI offer similar products!

A Quick Word About Nail Polish

Three ingredients have recently come under fire by a variety of groups promoting consumer safety: tuolamene, formaldehyde and DBP (Dibutyl Phthalate). All three of these ingredients have demonstrated the potential to cause sensitivity, allergic reactions or to be harmful to the human body. Yet, the FDA doesn't ban any of them[21] and the Nail Manufacturers Council of the Professional Beauty Association maintains that these ingredients are used in such small quantities as to be non-toxic and harmless.

However, in response to consumers' concerns, leading nail polish producers like OPI, Creative Nail Design, Zoya and Spa Ritual have abandoned the use of these ingredients (used to give the polish flexibility, sheen, hardness and consistent colour) in favour of other less toxic substances that provide the same finish.

One last tip: because anything applied to the nails keeps them from "breathing," it's very important to feed the cuticles and nail base with nail strengtheners to prevent them from splitting or becoming brittle. Most nail polish companies make them and your nail tech can recommend one for you.

What Makes a Good Manicure?

Like a pedicure, it is a straightforward procedure:

- Soaking the hands to soften the skin and cuticles,
- Cleaning the nails and pushing back the cuticles,
- Trimming the cuticles with special nippers or a liquid cuticle remover,
- Filing and shaping the nails,
- Massaging the hands and lower arms and
- Buffing and/or applying polish to the nails.

A spa manicure adds an exfoliating scrub, and often includes a paraffin dip or specialty wrap of some sort, as well as a more thorough hand and arm massage, making it a relaxing treatment rather than a purely "maintenance" service.

It should be noted that many spas have abandoned the use of nippers and scissors in favour of liquid cuticle removers that help soften the cuticles and slough the dead cells. This certainly cuts down on the risk of infection and makes it a safer procedure.

There's really not too much more to say — at least about nail care. Whether you opt for a spa manicure or pedicure — the first, optional for me, and the latter an absolute must — is for you to decide. The most important message in this chapter is that you pay scrupulous attention to the hygiene practices of the spa you do choose for these services — cheap can often equal somewhat less than clean and you may be putting yourself at risk for infection.

Having said all that, a pedicure is still one of my favourite treatments!

Chapter 11 Hair Today, Gone Tomorrow

Getting the Skinny on Hair Removal

This girl doesn't wax! Call me old school, but I hate the feel of stubble on my legs and would rather zip it off in the shower than wait to have it grow long enough to be pulled out by the roots once a month. And though laser hair removal is a distinct option, I just haven't got the patience.

However, I'm definitely in the minority! Waxing is the most popular service offered in most day spas today and laser hair removal is one of the hottest (no pun intended) growing treatments out there, so this topic deserves to be given more than just a quick once over.

Though waxing might seem pretty straightforward to most people, there are still a few do's and don'ts that are worth mentioning. And if some of this might seem a little intimate, it's because I've learned that waxing seems to go where the faint of heart dare not follow. It's also a heads up for you in case you're someone not familiar with every body part that can be waxed and who wants to know what to expect if you think you'd be a likely candidate.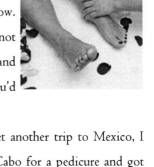

When in doubt, consult an expert, right? On yet another trip to Mexico, I stopped into a great little day spa in San Jose del Cabo for a pedicure and got into a great conversation with the owner, Kelli Castineiras, who has been in business for over ten years in this very busy tourist destination.

Since the sun almost always shines in this part of the world, there's a lot of exposed skin walking around that needs to look smooth and groomed (for gringos as well as locals), so waxing is a major part of her business. She had a lot of good advice that she was willing to share.

To Wax or Not to Wax

Pros

The part of your body that needs waxing is the issue. Facial waxing includes the eyebrows, upper lip, cheeks and chin. Body waxing includes the arms, legs, chest, bottom, back, bikini line and pubic area. One thing to consider with waxing is that some hair always grows back and to maintain the look and feel, you'll have to have follow-up treatments. But the hair regrowth in these areas tends to be reduced in quantity, lighter in colour and finer the more often you wax or sugar.

Cons

Waxing can be painful. After all, you are having the hair pulled out at the root. Depending on the density (number of hairs) and the coarseness of the hair, the procedures will be either more or less uncomfortable; but there are a number of steps, described later, that you can take to lessen the amount of discomfort.

You also must allow the hair to grow out before you can wax – to a minimum ¼ inch – in order for the wax to do its job effectively regardless of the part of the body being waxed. So you'll have to deal with the stubble!

How Hair Grows

Hair grows in three different cycles and at different rates. One hair may be in Cycle I while the one next to it is in Cycle II, so that in the process of hair removal (whether waxing, sugaring or laser) multiple treatments are necessary.

The myth that a hair removed grows back darker and coarser is just that – a myth. As noted above, regrowth may occur, but it's typically lighter and finer the more often you wax or sugar.

Legs, Chest, Back and Arms

Before beginning, your esthetician will cleanse the area and then apply talcum, oatmeal or a similar powder or protective oil to prevent the wax from sticking to the skin and pulling the skin off along with the hair. Then a comfortably hot wax is applied with a spatula or stick to the area about three inches wide and six inches long. As it hardens and envelops the hairs, a muslin strip is placed over the wax and, once cooled, is pulled off against the direction of hair growth in a smooth, quick motion. The esthetician will then rub the area gently and, once stray hairs have been tweezed and the entire area in question is finished, will apply an oatmeal or similar powder, oil or lotion to relieve any discomfort.

Face, Neck, Underarms, Bikini and Brazilian

These smaller areas tend to be more sensitive. A special hard wax is used for the process, in which the wax is first liquefied and applied at near body temperature. It is allowed to cool and set as it envelops the hairs and is then pulled off against the direction of hair growth, much like the cloth strips. And since wax can only be applied to an area once, any stray hairs will be tweezed away by the esthetician.

If you are prone to ingrown hairs, try gently exfoliating for the next couple of days after waxing and about once a week between waxing to keep the pores free of debris and the hairs pointing out and not curling back into the skin.

Brazilian Waxing

Brazilian waxing has become increasingly popular in the last few years. For some it's a matter of hygiene, for others a matter of personal esthetics because they prefer the "look," while for others it improves their more intimate relations with their partners.

There's absolutely no — well, very little - modesty allowed. After all, you have to lift your legs to your chest or spread them, so that the service provider can work on the areas involved. Many places encourage you to feel as comfortable as possible and don't mind if you leave your panties on or will provide a paper panty or thong if you'd like, but the esthetician still has to move the panty over, so what's the point? Speaking of which, the hair should be trimmed to about ¼" for fine hair and a ½" for coarser hair which will cut down on the amount of sensitivity/pain involved, especially the first time.

As to how much hair is left, you have the choice of having all of it removed or leaving a narrow "landing" strip, a small triangle of hair or even a design. Again, it's a personal preference.

The wax is applied in the direction of the hair growth and then stripped away "against the grain" in one long, smooth motion. Your service provider will need to place her hand on your labia in order to hold the skin firmly enough to pull out the hairs or she might ask you to help. Most estheticians advocate the use of a hard wax that doesn't require strips (Kelli says she only uses high quality hard wax to get the best results and cut down on irritation or sensitivity – especially post-waxing – and uses the wax only for that particular person for hygienic and safety reasons). If you're not sure about your spa's practices, ask, and if it is used multiple times, then double dipping is absolutely forbidden.

Waxing the genital area in both men and women can also include the area around the anus, so be specific with your service provider as to what hair you want removed from front to back.

Sugaring

Sugaring is very similar to waxing but is somewhat gentler on the skin in that it attaches to only the hair and any residue on the skin can be easily washed off. It is applied at room temperature, thus eliminating the chance of burning the skin, and unlike waxes does not adhere to live skin cells (only to dead ones) making it an exfoliant at the same time. Cloth strips are applied to the sugar, water and lemon juice paste and pulled off in the direction of the hair growth. The hair only needs to be 1/16" long and for sensitive skin sugaring is considered a good alternative to waxing.

Many spas use a sugar gel rather than a paste and call it sugar waxing. The gel has many of the same properties as wax in that the hair needs to be ¼" long and is applied and removed the same way as in waxing. It is said to also have the same drawbacks – like ingrown hairs, irritation and broken hairs. So be sure to check which version of the two treatments is meant when the spa offers sugaring on its menu.

Threading

This is an ancient technique involving a fine thread that is looped around one or more hairs that is then pulled tight, removing the hairs from the follicles. It is performed incredibly fast and used primarily for the eyebrows and other facial hair. Many people prefer it saying that it gives a smoother look and allows the brows to be perfectly shaped. Like sugaring, it's not a service commonly found in most spas, but go online for one near you and give it a try.

 Waxing and Teens

After my 14 year-old granddaughter went to a spa to have her legs waxed, we started talking about the service. Much to my surprise (she lives in San Jose, CA), she had been having waxing services for the last two years. It all started with her "uni-brow" and progressed from there – especially as she's a swimmer and swims and plays water polo competitively. When I asked her if there were any drawbacks, she replied, "It hurts!" She went on to say, though, that it's definitely worth it. Would she recommend it for other teens?

"Yes! Because I don't need to shave as often between times and it seems like there's less hair growth."

Waxing Do's and Don't's

There are a number of things you can do to ensure that your waxing experience is worth it and produces optimal results:

Do: take an ibuprofen or two – especially for waxing in the bikini
        area – 30 minutes to an hour before your appointment.

Do: wait for a week after your period to have a Brazilian or bikini to reduce sensitivity in the area.

Do: apply an antibacterial lotion to the waxed area afterward, being very careful around the sensitive genital area, since the pores and follicles are open and susceptible to infection.

Do: avoid caffeine and alcohol for at least 2-3 hours before waxing, as that increases the body's acidity which heightens sensitivity; instead hydrate with plenty of water.

Do: gently exfoliate before waxing to remove dead skin and debris in the pores that can keep the hairs from being easily removed.

Do: go to a reputable spa and make sure that your esthetician has experience in the particular technique you're looking for.

Don't: vigorously exfoliate the area for at least 24 hours afterwards.

Don't: expose the area to the sun for 24 hours prior to waxing and 48 hours thereafter.

Don't: apply any astringents, toners or ice prior to the treatment because they cause the pores to constrict and you want them nice and relaxed so that the hairs can be removed more easily.

Don't: apply lotions or oils to the skin on the same day as your treatment (except for an antibacterial lotion afterwards).

Don't: go to a spa that double dips or that is less than spotlessly clean.

Waxing Alert!

Are you taking any medications such as Accutane, Retinol, Retin A or others that cause the skin to thin or become more sensitive? If you are or have taken them within the past 12 months, don't wax!

As a matter of fact, waxing is not recommended for anyone with thin or weak skin because it can lead to tearing and possible infection. Please check with your doctor before considering waxing, especially if you use steroid creams and medications or have diabetes. And be sure to ask your service provider while having a chemical peel or laser treatment as to when you can resume waxing.

If you have varicose veins or moles and skin tags, the wax should not be applied to those areas. And, of course, if you have allergies to any of the ingredients, waxing is to be avoided.

The Beauty of Laser and IPL Hair Removal

It really does depend upon the amount of body and facial hair you have and its colour. Although fair skinned persons with dark hair are terrific candidates for laser hair removal, blondes and redheads are less so and those with grey hair are not due to the lack of melanin in their hair that attracts the laser beam that then destroys the hair follicle.

Although not the case a few years ago, dark skin types now can have unwanted hair removed safely through the use of ND:YAG lasers; however, Intense Pulsed Light (IPL) can cause problems like irritation and even damage the skin. The process itself may also take longer or require a greater number of treatments. If this could be you, please consult a medical spa or dermatologist to ensure that the proper equipment and number of treatments are appropriate for you to avoid burning and scarring of your skin.

As the laser passes over the skin, each hair absorbs the intense light down into the follicle that is then disabled or destroyed. Remember how hair grows in stages or cycles? Some of the hairs are bound to be dormant or invisible and so won't be affected by the laser or IPL during your treatment. As a result, it can take several months and from 6-10 treatments to see an up to 90-95% reduction. As for laser therapy, the FDA has only approved the descriptor "hair reduction" as opposed to "permanent hair removal" because there can always be some re-growth.

But beware! The terms laser and intense pulsed light (IPL) are often used interchangeably and though both can be effective, you'll need to be careful when selecting your service provider. Personally, I would not consider a spa that is not operated under the direct supervision of a medical doctor.

For most women, and a lot of men, getting rid of unwanted hair is an ongoing, never ending battle. Of course you can wax at home yourself or even find what you're looking for in a salon, but it's only at a spa that your service can become more than just a service…except for some forms of waxing! Brazilian, anyone?

Chapter 12 Is the Doctor In? Medical Spas

Boomers are hitting their 50's and 60's in droves; their influence and impact as consumers undiminished as they age. They are part of a Mainstream (North) America that continues its ever-present search for the fountain of youth, personified by Hollywood glam and fueled by reality shows and slick fashion mags.

Not surprisingly, the number of people north and south of the border looking for a nip here and a tuck there continues to grow. But not everyone is interested in cosmetic surgery to achieve his or her esthetic goals and, as a consequence, medical spas have also continued to increase in popularity.

The Medical Spa Explosion

In the past five years, I have seen the number of medical spas in my area double in number – with general practitioners, plastic surgeons, dermatologists and dental centres adding treatments like Botox®; fillers like Juvederm and Restylane; photorejuvenation; laser hair removal and a number of other equally interesting treatments to their practices. Everyone, it seems, is jumping on the anti-aging, "look good" bandwagon.

This phenomenon can be found in cities large and small as more and more men and women opt to do something about their looks rather than sitting idly by and letting time take its toll. Whether this is simply a Boomer phenomenon or is due to the significant advances in technology that have made medical esthetic treatments accessible to the average consumer is a good question. Probably both, since the past decade saw an unprecedented rise in the number of medical spas (83% of all medical spas in the U.S. started up after the year 2000).

Maybe you, too, have been considering having unwanted facial and body hair removed with precision, getting a "fix" for your drooping eyelids, tightening loose skin or plumping up your lips (to name only a few of the many procedures available), but aren't sure whether to opt for plastic surgery or try something less invasive. Perhaps a consultation at a medical spa near you is the answer.

The Medical Spa Defined

If you're not quite sure what qualifies as a medical spa, the International Spa Association defines it as:

> "A facility that operates under the full-time, on-site supervision of a licensed health care professional whose primary purpose is to provide comprehensive medical and wellness care in an environment that integrates spa services, as well as traditional, complimentary and/or alternative therapies and treatments. The facility operates within the scope of practice of its staff, which can include both aesthetic/cosmetic and prevention/wellness procedures and services."

The Canadians go a little further and their national spa association, Spa Industry Association of Canada, states:

> "The practitioner must be a licensed medical doctor with a valid College of Physicians and Surgeons Registration for the province in which treatments are offered. The physician must also be a current member of the Canadian Medical Protective Association and have informed the CMPA in writing of their provision of the medical aesthetic procedures and/or a registered nurse with valid registration with the Nursing Association for the province in which treatments are offered. For nurses providing services, a licensed medical doctor with valid College of Physician and Surgeons registration must supervise the procedures."

As a rule, medical spas offer non-surgical procedures that make use of advanced technologies and medical or pharmaceutical-grade products which treat the skin more intensively than standard spa treatments. Although these procedures are non-surgical, some can still be so highly intensive that they require many days of downtime while your skin heals.

Because there are so many different medical aesthetic options available today, the invaluable guidance of an experienced physician can make all the difference in achieving your goals, whatever they may be. A physician with training in aesthetic medicine will be able to ensure that your course of treatment is appropriate to you and deal with any side effects or complications that might arise. Be aware that in the hands of providers who lack the knowledge, experience or training necessary to safely administer treatments that are really effective, you can wind up with scarring and other unwanted results – including no results at all. So, keep in mind that even though you might think you're spending more in a reputable medical spa, in the long run you'll probably end up spending less.

Many medical spas also offer traditional skin care and nail services, as well as lifestyle and/or complementary therapies, found in "regular" spas. And interestingly, 15% of non-medical spas offer medically supervised services ranging from Botox® and fillers to microdermabrasion to chemical peels. Optimally, this means that a licensed health care professional comes to the spa on a predetermined basis and provides these treatments or supervises their application by other licensed individuals, but unfortunately this is not always the case.

Top 5 Questions to Ask Before Booking a Medical Aesthetics Procedure

Would you take your toaster to a plumber to repair it? No? Well, why would you allow someone without the necessary years of experience and credentialed training to inject your Botox® or perform photorejuvenation on your face?

Unless you've booked an esthetics treatment, such as a pedicure, that you can find at a "regular" spa (provided that the medical spa in question even offers such treatments), it is especially critical when considering any procedure requiring

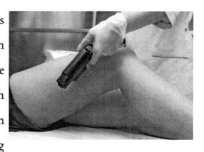

penetration or removal of the epidermis, including injections or laser therapies, that you schedule an interview with your medical spa or treatment centre and ask the questions suggested below:

I. Who will perform the procedure and what are his or her qualifications?

A weekend course in the operation of a particular piece of equipment or administration of Botox® and dermal fillers does not necessarily mean that the person performing your procedure has the understanding, knowledge, expertise or experience to provide your desired results or deal with any complications that might arise.

For some of the more invasive procedures, such as deep chemical peels and certain laser treatments, it is highly recommended that you seek out a dermatologist or plastic surgeon. If there should be complications, these board-certified specialists are in a position to handle them.

At the very least, your medical spa should operate under the direct supervision of a medical doctor. Ensure that the doctor is on site and present – some laser centres and "medi-spas" operate under a "medical director" that may not be available if something should go wrong.

2. How often has the doctor or his staff performed this procedure?

Just because the doctor has a medical background, does not mean that he or she has the training for such procedures as injectables like

Botox® or fillers like Restylane or Juvederm. The doctor should administer them on a regular basis.

Medical spa staff such as Registered Nurses and Professional Assistants will usually perform procedures like laser hair removal, microdermabrasion, mild to moderate chemical peels and advanced aesthetic treatments for acne, rosacea and anti-aging. In some medical spas, RN's have also been trained to administer injectables, so be sure to ask about their credentials and how much experience they have in the particular treatment you want and with your particular skin type.

If you have further questions or concerns, you should be able to address them with the Medical Doctor in charge. Conversely, if the medical spa can't or won't accommodate you, move on and consult the web sites listed in the Resource Guide or a dermatologist to find a qualified provider in your area before exposing yourself to unnecessary risks.

3. *May I see before and after photos of patients and/or read testimonials or speak with former clients?*

If the medical spa can't or won't share this information, go elsewhere.

4. *Will there be an initial consultation?*

A consultation is an absolute prerequisite to any medical cosmetic procedure, regardless of its intensity. Whether it is conducted by the person who will perform the procedure or not, it should include your complete medical history and include a discussion that covers the following:

• What you specifically want to achieve with your visit: tighten the skin under your eyes, firm sagging jowls, remove age spots, firm a sagging tummy, smooth the wrinkles in your forehead, remove spider veins, etc.

- The type and frequency of the procedure (or a combination of techniques if indicated) required to achieve your desired results, what these results will be and whether your expectations are reasonable, achievable and appropriate to your age, health and lifestyle.

- Where and how the equipment will be used on you or where the injections will be placed and who will be performing the procedure.

- Cost per unit or type of treatment, how many units or treatments will be required in total and how payment will be made (insurance doesn't normally cover such procedures). Some courses of treatment can easily run to several thousand dollars!

- What risks and/or side effects may be involved (and be advised that there are risks associated with these treatments that need to be addressed and acknowledged).

- What follow-up care is required and how long it will take – some procedures cause scabbing, redness and a good deal of pain and require prolonged after-care. Be sure it's worth it to you and whether there may be alternative medical aesthetic procedures that can achieve similar results.

- How long before you'll see results and how long the results will last.

5. *What skin care regimen do you recommend before, during and after the treatment (or series of treatments) to achieve and maintain my goals?*

   Obviously, prior preparation and a good home maintenance program will ensure that you maximize the benefits of the treatments or procedures that you have decided to undergo – not to mention the money that you are investing in enhancing your appearance or correcting flaws or problems that have plagued you in the past.

So What's the Diff? Isn't a Doctor a Doctor?

We know that a medical spa must be under the direct supervision of an MD, but which discipline? Today, you'll find general practitioners, dentists, dermatologists and plastic surgeons offering many of the same procedures. So who is qualified to do what?

General Practitioners – are qualified medical doctors, having completed four years of medical school, in addition to four years of university, and an additional 2-6 years in residency; may be excellent cosmetic specialists as a result of years of experience and additional training, but are not recommended for many of the specialized laser, deep chemical peels or other advanced procedures that are the purview of dermatologists or cosmetic surgeons.

Dentists – have completed 2-4 years of college or university pre-dental education, followed by four years at an accredited dental school; have good knowledge of the lower part of the face, but in general have no specialized training in the skin and muscles of the upper face. Although currently approved to provide Botox® and injectables in nearly half the United States and some Canadian provinces primarily for dental conditions such as TMD, the debate continues between the medical and dental community as to whether dentists have the training necessary to provide cosmetic treatments and deal with potential complications.

Dermatologists – are medical doctors with an additional five years of specialized study of the skin; are required to maintain their credentials with advanced yearly training; can provide a wider selection of technologies devoted to non-surgical medical aesthetics and can best recognize and recommend the most appropriate procedures for dealing with specific conditions or areas of the face and body and remedy any complications that might arise.

Plastic Surgeons – are medical doctors with five additional years of surgical training including two years of specific training in plastic surgery (required for members of the American Society for Aesthetic Plastic Surgery); are generally focused on surgery to correct cosmetic concerns/conditions found in the face and body, rather than non-surgical procedures that work within the dermis and epidermis to improve a person's appearance, but may also provide non-surgical medical aesthetic procedures in their practices.

According to Dr. Wendy Smeltzer, M.D., C.C.F.P., F.C.F.P., founder of Canada's first medical spa and board member of the Canadian Association of Aesthetic Medicine, the future of aesthetic/cosmetic medicine is beginning to look a little brighter from the consumer's perspective. CAAM is currently developing a standardized training program in Aesthetic Medicine for physicians from all disciplines who wish to offer medical aesthetics.

"Right now," says Dr. Smeltzer, "there is no assurance that just because it is a physician offering these services that they have expertise in that area. There are some dermatologists who have intensive knowledge of diseases of the skin and some plastic surgeons with their extensive surgical skills who have no formal training in administering Botox® and other injectables or providing laser treatments, not to mention other MD's and dentists that are adding medical aesthetics to their practices who have little knowledge or training in this field."

Aesthetic Medicine in the United States and Canada is not yet a recognized medical specialty and as a result is largely unregulated in terms of standards for accreditation and certification for the competent provision of the technologies available today – including injectables. Consequently, developing a standardized aesthetic medical training program for physicians across the board, regardless of their specialty, would take much of the guesswork out of the consumer's quest for expert aesthetic medical service providers.

When you find medically-based treatments like microdermabrasion or laser hair removal at your corner spa, be careful, do your homework and make sure that you're not letting yourself in for problems and a waste of your hard-earned money down the road. The range of equipment available to these non-medical individuals and/or spas is not as intensive as you would find in a physician's practice and might not be as effective from a cost or results perspective.

And if you have the option of having Botox® or injectables in a home or at a party, just know that it is not only considered unethical by the medical community, it carries real risk or potential danger for you!

Botox® and Other Injectables

Botox® is a prescription drug approved by the FDA and by Health Canada specifically for the treatment of cervical dystonia and frown lines between the eyebrows, but is also typically used for crows feet, horizontal lines on the forehead, lines on the neck, lifting the brow and shaping the eyebrow. It works by blocking the messages transmitted by the nerves to the muscles that cause them to contract and move. Botox® can have side effects and must be given in an environment where any complications that arise can be dealt with immediately and professionally.

Did you get that? Botox® is a *prescription drug*. It is sold by its producer, Allergan, only to medical doctors. Although there are other botulinium-A products available, such as Dysport, Xeomin and Myobloc, Botox® is the one still most commonly administered for cosmetic purposes.

Botox® parties? Self injections? Would you buy a prescription-only, heavy-duty painkiller from a dealer on the street? Botox® is a drug sold to MD's – purely and simply – and intended for use by them or under their direct supervision. And unfortunately there are now knock-offs offered by unethical providers that can be downright dangerous, so ensure your provider is using legitimate Botox® (the bottle has a hologram on it).

Since these injections require a *precise knowledge* of facial anatomy, your risk of complications increases when Botox® injections are performed by unskilled injectors. Your provider must possess the skill and expertise to select the correct injection points and/or proper dosages, in order to avoid unwanted results. A thorough understanding of the interaction and interdependency of the muscles of the face is imperative.

This is equally important in injecting fillers like Juvederm and Restylane that are used to add volume to the areas in and around wrinkles, folds and depressions of nearly every area of the face. Fillers are also used for the hands, injected under the balls of the feet to lessen pain from high heels and for improving the appearance of scars.

Those in the know maintain that providing Botox® and other injectables is one part science and the other part art. Even within the medical community, there are good and bad providers. There are some RN's who have the expertise and skill of an experienced MD and some doctors that you wouldn't want to let near you. Find a physician that understands you and your needs and that has the experience and judgment to see exactly what he or she must do to enhance your looks most effectively.

The bottom line? Do your homework. Listen to your friends or family members and ask the questions listed above. Check with your local and state or provincial medical boards as to their qualifications and credentials.

To find out more, check the Resource Guide under Medical Aesthetics at the end of the book. The producers of Botox® also provide a list of approved doctors at www.botoxcosmetic.com and www.botoxcosmetic.ca. An excellent publication that I highly recommend is <u>New Beauty Magazine</u>, published quarterly, www.newbeauty.com, for the latest and most up to date information on a wide range of beauty and medical aesthetics issues.

When Should You Consider Visiting a Medical Spa?

At some point it may be that your "regular" spa just can't provide the results you're looking for and the more advanced procedures found in a medical spa could be the answer.

Dull and lifeless skin; fine lines and wrinkles; scarring from acne or getting rid of pesky age spots might be a starting point. There are a number of other cosmetic concerns that might seem trivial to others but important to you, so why "grin and bear it" when you can do something about them?

Perhaps the most important question to ask yourself is whether you are willing to invest the time and money needed to produce optimum results. These procedures are not quick fixes for the most part. Many require a series of treatments or, as in the case of most injectables, may only last for a relatively limited time and need further treatments to maintain your desired outcome. It all depends on what you want to accomplish.

 ## Medical vs. Non-medical Spas and Treatment Centres

Buyer beware! Inexperienced, poorly trained technicians in a non-medical spa or "laser" centre can turn your "photofacial," IPL hair removal, cellulite treatment, microdermabrasion or chemical peel into your worst nightmare! These treatments are serious and require the eye and expertise of a qualified, experienced Medical Doctor or his Registered Nurse or Physician's Assistant in order to assess and provide the best type of equipment and/or procedure for you.

There are so many different kinds of equipment on the market today that it makes your head spin. Choosing the right one can only be done after a thorough diagnosis of your skin and lifestyle – something most technicians don't possess the knowledge or skill to make. You can wind up with complications like scarring from burns and changes in pigmentation on the one hand to lousy results on the other. Talk to a dermatologist and he or she will tell you that they see the results of badly done treatments on the average of once a week.

In the case of more advanced medical aesthetics, including laser treatments like Fraxl, Thermage, intense chemical peels, etc. that work in the deeper levels of the skin, please choose the medical spa of an experienced medical doctor, dermatologist or plastic surgeon who has experience with these procedures after doing your research. Depending on the intensity and type of treatment, ask for references and how long he or she has practiced medical aesthetics.

The upshot? Don't base your decision on the spa or laser centre's hype or price. It's just not worth it!

Medical Aesthetic Treatments Explained

For each of the following, there are variations in the types of equipment from low to high end as well as differences in the technologies themselves. And by the time you read this, there will most certainly be new, exciting advanced treatments and technologies to add to the list below.

Most of the treatments and procedures can be found in a typical medical spa, but not all. It depends on the level of training and expertise of the particular Medical Doctor and/or his or her staff.

Your age along with the amount of collagen still present in your skin; the amount of sun damage you have experienced; the colour of your skin; scarring; medical conditions such as acne and rosacea and other factors must be considered by the spa's medical professionals when recommending a course of treatment for you. There is no "one size fits all" approach and what was great for your best friend might be completely wrong for you.

Microdermabrasion: tiny grains of aluminum oxide, a diamond tipped head or infrared light are passed over the surface of the skin by means of a small wand and simultaneously vacuumed up along with the surface dead skin cells that are loosened in a process akin to sanding the skin. Multiple treatments may be necessary before the desired results are achieved. Recommended for mild acne scars, age spots, sun-damaged skin, fine lines and wrinkles, minimizing skin pore size, rejuvenating skin tone and improving skin texture.

Chemical peels: can be superficial, medium or deep with appropriate post-treatments and recovery procedures for each. Chemicals applied to the skin remove damaged skin cells at different levels: deep peels require general anesthesia, can cause scabs to form and involve extensive post-treatment procedures lasting 14-21 days. You'll find glycolic acid, hydroxy acid and vitamin treatments (up to 20%) in regular spas for superficial peels, but for medium to deep peels, a specialist (dermatologist or plastic surgeon) is required. Recommended for a dull complexion, to remove fine lines and wrinkles, remove acne scars and improve skin texture.

Botox®: the botulinum toxin in this approved form is generally injected into the muscles of the face that cause frown lines and crow's feet and effectively immobilizes them for up to 4-6 months. It is also used to address excessive underarm perspiration. There can be side effects and it is recommended that only medical professionals provide injections. Not administered to patients under18 years of age. Also check to see when the Botox® was diluted with saline solution and if it is refrigerated (many MDs report that once diluted, it is effective for up to two weeks thereafter if kept refrigerated). See the Botox® web site for more information.

Fillers: both permanent (less common) and non-permanent (absorbed by the body over time) are used to add volume to the areas in and around wrinkles, folds and depressions of nearly every area of the face, also the hands, under the balls of the feet to ease the pain of high heels and for improving the appearance of scars. Permanent fillers include polymethylmethacrylate (PMMA) that is a suspension of synthetic polymere beads or microspheres in several different colloids such as bovine collagen or hyaluronic acid. Different types of non-permanent include collagen derived from human, bovine and pig sources; a variety of hyaluronic acid brands or using a person's own body fat. They last usually 3-4 months, although the pig-based collagen can last up to 12 months. Good for plumping lips, filling out hollow cheeks, improving scars, elevating deep folds and repairing various facial imperfections.

Hair removal can be applied to any part of the body and is particularly effective for lighter skin with darker hairs. The pigment in the hair absorbs the laser or IPL converting it to heat and disabling the hair follicle. Unlike electrolysis, it covers a larger area of the skin and more hairs. Blondes, redheads, and dark or deeply tanned skin should consult a medical doctor or dermatologist before beginning a course of treatment to avoid blistering, burning or other potential problems. Can be Intense Pulsed Light or Laser and may require multiple treatments. Some hair may regrow.

Laser skin treatments include ablative (removes the stratum corneum or top layer of the skin and stimulates the growth of new collagen in the dermis) or non-ablative and fractionated (leaves the stratum corneum intact while penetrating to the dermis below). Ablative lasers include er:YAGs and carbon dioxide lasers that produce dramatic results. Non-ablative include fractional, ND:YAG, thermage (radio frequency) and even cold-based lasers. Results with non-ablatives tend to be gradual and can require multiple treatments for the desired effect. Your dermatologist or plastic surgeon can recommend the most appropriate treatment type for you. Lasers stimulate new collagen production in the dermis, reduce cellulite, tighten skin, smooth texture, reduce wrinkles and scarring and even remove tattoos.

Intense Pulsed Light (IPL) therapy: (non ablative and not a laser), often referred to as photorejuvenation, in which pulses of non-coherent, wide-spectrum light are flashed through a glass prism placed over the skin after a cold gel is applied to the area to be treated. The light is absorbed by the targeted tissue and leaves the surrounding tissue intact with minimal downtime, compared to some chemical peels and laser treatments, and usually only creates a mild redness that should quickly disappear. Not recommended for dark or deeply tanned skin; within 6 months of discontinuing use of Accutane or for pregnant women. Recommended for reducing age spots, discolorations and rosacea and generally requires a series of 3-5 treatments over a specific time period. Skin tightening is minimal.

LED Light: known as photo biomodulation, using both red and infrared technology that stimulates the skin to heal itself; reduces redness as a result of cosmetic procedures such as chemical peels, IPL photofacials, medical microdermabrasion and even sunburn.

Radio Frequency treatments: (non-ablative) known as Thermage that tightens and contours lax skin by stimulating collagen production through pulses of radio-frequency energy deep into the dermis. It helps tighten loose skin around the lower face and jawline, but is also considered effective in treating cellulite and the neck, eyes, arms, buttocks, thighs and tummy.

Cosmetic Dentistry: basically any treatment or work that improves the appearance and/or function of the teeth, including crowns; whitening treatments including blue light and laser; implants and veneers; contouring of the teeth and invisible braces. Look for dentists who are members of the American Academy of Cosmetic Dentistry, including Canadian cosmetic dentists.

Cosmeceuticals: are advanced skin care lines available at medical spas to enhance the efficacy of the treatments provided. Medical spa staff can make the appropriate recommendations. Certain lines are not carried in regular spas and are only available at medical spas.

What's Your Follow-through I.Q.?

For most of these treatment/procedures, you'll have to do your part to make sure that you achieve the results you want:

- Follow the home care directions of your doctor to the letter – if you need to cool your face every 20 minutes, do it! Do you need to apply a cream or lotion? Do it diligently.

- If you smoke, don't do it during your recovery period! Smoking deprives the tissues of oxygen and slows wound healing.

- Wear 30+ SPF full-spectrum sunscreen after any procedure involving the epidermis or dermal layer as soon as indicated by your physician before going out in the sun. Your epidermis has been compromised and needs the protection.

If you think I'm being a little too cautious in recommending that these treatments only be performed by a medical doctor or under the direct supervision of a trained MD, check this out: in a survey performed in 2007 by the American Society for Dermatologic Surgery, 56% of the dermatologic surgeons reported that they are treating more and more patients for complications from cosmetic procedures like chemical peels and laser therapy performed by non-physicians.

What to Do if There's No Medical Spa Near You

If you live in an area where there is no medical spa available, but there is a doctor or dentist or possibly a spa offering microdermabrasion, laser treatments and injectables, please, please be careful and do your homework. Be absolutely brazen and ask where they have trained and who will be providing your chosen service within the practice. Injectables, especially, have become a cash cow for many dentists and doctors. The same holds true for spas offering these procedures in foreign countries.

Also, keep in mind when traveling outside of your home area that in order for you to achieve your desired results, a single treatment might not be sufficient and multiple treatments might be necessary. Will you be in the vicinity of your provider long enough to take care of any complications that might arise or to see your treatments through? Checking the qualifications of your provider could also prove challenging.

Is a medical spa for you? The money and time that you are prepared to invest in improving your appearance is a decision that only you can make. But once you have made the commitment, a medical aesthetics specialist can help you look more youthful and feel more self-assured. Join the hundreds of thousands of men and women who have found out for themselves!

Chapter 13 Spas and Wellness

Benjamin Franklin said it more than 200 years ago, "An ounce of prevention is worth a pound of cure," and millions of North Americans still continue to take his timeless advice, embracing wellness in its many forms for a more proactive approach to achieving and maintaining good health.

Why include a chapter on wellness in a 'How-to" book on spa going? The better you understand the *concept* of wellness, the easier it will be to make sense of the ways the term is being broadly used in the media, in advertising, within the medical community and especially in the spa.

Spas provide many of the tools that can help you enjoy an active, healthy life, such as yoga, exercise, meditation, aromatherapy, massage, hydrotherapy, nutritional counselling and stress management, all of which are important facets of the wellness spectrum.

First, we'll define wellness, see how spa relates to wellness as a whole and then examine how so many of the wellness therapies found in complementary and alternative medicine have assured their place in an integrative health care model.

Next, we'll look at three major factors that have come together to precipitate a shift from reactive (sole reliance on conventional medicine) towards proactive (wellness-related) health care and finish up with a report from the 2011 Global Spa Summit on Wellness Tourism.

It's a lot of information, I know, but it underscores the important roles spas and wellness play in supporting us as we take responsibility for our own personal health and wellbeing.

Wellness Defined

We need to clearly define the term and then examine how and where spa fits into the wellness spectrum.

In the preamble to the Constitution of the World Health Organization written in 1948, "health" was defined as *a state of complete physical, mental and social wellbeing and not merely the absence of disease or infirmity.*

The actual term "wellness" was first coined by physician Halbert L. Dunn in his 1961 book, *High-Level Wellness*, and wasn't really picked up again until after the world's first wellness establishment, the Wellness Resource Center in Mill Valley, CA, was opened by Dr. John Travis in 1975. The term really caught on, however, after Paul Zane Pilzer's book, *The Wellness Revolution*, hit the newsstands in 2002 where he described wellness as an industry, predicting it would be "the next Trillion Dollar Industry."

He wasn't far off the mark. The wellness industry has become firmly established worldwide and in 2010 was estimated to be worth $2 trillion dollars with 289 million wellness consumers in the top 30 wealthiest, industrialized countries.

In the context of this chapter, let us agree that wellness can be defined as a *complete state in which an individual assumes responsibility for his or her personal lifestyle and health by making positive decisions in regards to social, emotional, economic, environmental, physical and spiritual alternatives. It is not just the absence of disease.*

It's still a fairly broad interpretation, but stays within the parameters of taking a "proactive" and holistic approach, as well as personal responsibility, for our individual health and wellbeing.

Spas as Part of the Wellness Spectrum

Since by definition wellness encompasses the totality of a person's health and wellbeing, it meshes nicely with Spa's emphasis on mind, body and spirit. Touch in its many forms helps the body either regain or maintain vitality, just as meditation or yoga helps you clear your mind and restore your inner balance. So, by visiting a spa, you are taking a proactive step in positively influencing the state of your physical, mental and emotional health.

From this perspective, you begin to see how spas fit into the wellness picture. History tends to come full circle and perhaps the resurgence of spas in the last several decades was inevitable as people sought alternate ways to revitalize, restore and improve their wellbeing. The difference between now and yesteryear is that while spas once were places where people sought cures for the illnesses of the body, today's spas tend to provide respite from stress and the ever-increasing demands and immediacy of our technology-driven society.

And where water was once the focal point of spa culture, the majority of today's spas are defined by the healing power of touch in its many forms. Though still an integral part of many spas, water now shares in importance with lifestyle programs and fitness, trailing behind esthetics and massage.

As you look more closely, you realize that these are key elements in the wellness spectrum. The beauty is that rather than searching out different sources to find and take advantage of these many modalities, spas can provide an accessible "one stop shop" for the savvy consumer.

For decades, wellness has been at the core of most destination spas (and some resort and day spas) in the form of counselling, fitness, nutrition and lifestyle programs. And some, such as Canyon Ranch, Miraval, Red Mountain Resort, The Marsh, The Raj Ayurveda Health Spa, The Pritikin Longevity Center and Cooper Fitness Spa, have medical personnel on staff, incorporating medical testing and analyses not only for people with issues such as weight, sleep and stress-related problems (and even certain medical issues) but also for active, healthy clients and guests who want to stay that way.

As the spa community gravitates toward a more wellness-based focus and reaches out to the millions of health and wellness consumers worldwide, you will find more and more spas' treatment menus, brochures, web sites, advertising and public relations efforts reflecting the wellness message with a more targeted and specific approach.

For many, the concept of Spa has been synonymous with pampering and self-indulgence. Have you, too, struggled with this idea? What, then, can account for the unabated growth of the spa industry? It is a result, I am convinced, of the profound desire so many people have for a more nurturing and compassionate means of "taking care of" themselves.

Stop and consider that what you might believe to be pampering most probably has a significantly positive impact on your physical and emotional wellbeing. Can you think of a more enjoyable way of keeping healthy? Didn't think so.

Wellness and Medicine – Compatible or Not?

The following is my personal assessment of the wellness/conventional medicine situation at the present. Keep in mind that this is not a scientific analysis, but drawn from my own years of research and experience. I invite you to learn as much as you can about this topic, judge for yourself and draw your own conclusions.

To administer medicines to diseases which have already developed and thereby suppress bodily chaos which has already occurred is comparable to the behavior of those who would begin to dig a well after they have grown thirsty, or those who would begin to cast weapons after they have engaged in battle. Would these actions not be too late?

- From The Yellow Emperor's Inner
Medicine Classic, 500 B.C.

Integrative, Complementary and Alternative Medicine on the Rise

Conventional, mainstream medicine reacts to (and treats and cures) existing symptoms and conditions of sickness in a variety of ways using a variety of means. Wellness takes a proactive approach, keeping a person healthy by means of a diverse range of goods and services aimed at the prevention of sickness and slowing the effects of aging, often employing CAM therapies that cross over into both categories.

An approach that combines the two is slowly becoming more prevalent with clinics integrating conventional, mainstream medicine and complementary therapies, known as integrative medicine, defined below. An excellent list of therapies more commonly used in integrative medicine clinics and centers can be found on the Bravewell Collaborative site.

Definitions

First of all, it's important to understand the difference between healing and curing. Healing can be defined as producing a harmony of mind, body and spirit. A person may be "cured" of a disease, but still be angry, filled with despair or unable to function properly. True healing comes when body, mind and spirit have come into balance.

Both integrative medicine and complementary and alternative medicine (CAM) go beyond traditional curing to integrating emotional and spiritual well-being into the healing process, but there are important differences between them.

According to the National Center for Complementary and Alternative medicine at the National Institutes of Health:

- Integrative medicine combines treatments from conventional medicine and CAM for which there is evidence of safety and effectiveness. It is also called integrated medicine.

- Complementary medicine is used together with conventional medicine. An example of a complementary therapy is using acupuncture in addition to usual care to help lessen pain.
- Alternative medicine is used in place of conventional medicine.[22]

This is perhaps the best available definition:

"Integrative Medicine is the practice of medicine that reaffirms the importance of the relationship between practitioner and patient, focuses on the whole person, is informed by evidence, and makes use of all appropriate therapeutic approaches, healthcare professionals and disciplines to achieve optimal health and healing."

- Developed and Adopted by the Consortium of Academic Health Centers for Integrative Medicine, May 2004, Edited May 2009[23]

The American Hospital Association (AHA) Health Forum/Samueli Institute 2010 Complementary and Alternative Medicine Survey of Hospitals, released September 2011, showed that more than 42% of responding hospitals indicated they offer one or more CAM therapies (up from 37% percent in 2007). According to the survey, 85% of the hospitals indicated patient demand as the primary rationale in offering CAM services and 70% of survey respondents stated clinical effectiveness in selecting the CAM therapies they offer. Massage therapy was in the top two in- and out-patient services offered and, interestingly, most of the CAM services provided were not reimbursable by insurance and were paid for out-of-pocket by the patients.

The study notes that "Researchers at the University of California, Los Angeles, and the University of California, San Diego, measured medical students' attitudes and beliefs about CAM and found that three-quarters of them felt conventional Western medicine would benefit by integrating more CAM therapies and ideas."

It also mentions a 2009 Survey of Health Care Consumers conducted by Deloitte in which it was reported that the American public spent approximately $12–19 billion on CAM providers and a total of $36–47 billion on all services and products combined.[24]

The Bravewell Collaborative captured the spirit of tomorrow's integrated medical approach to health care most succinctly when it created the "Patient's Bill of Rights." It states that:

As an individual, you have:

- The right to person-centered care.
- The right to receive health care that addresses the wholeness of who you are – body, mind and spirit in the context of community.
- The right to a health care system that focuses on prevention and wellness.
- The right to be empowered as the responsible, central actor in your own healing.
- The right to education about self-care that includes access to scientifically-based nutrition, exercise and mind-body interventions.
- The right to a healing relationship with your health care provider that is grounded in humanism, compassion and caring.
- The right to speak openly and honestly with your health care providers and in return, to experience honest and supportive communications from all members of the health care community.
- The right to a health care environment that recognizes that to be healing and empowering, health care providers themselves must seek to be restored and whole.
- The right to embrace the spiritual dimension in the context of your health care.

- The right to health care providers who understand that integrity and spiritual qualities are as important as medical knowledge and technical skills in the process of healing.

- The right to a truly integrative medicine that is supported by rigorous scientific research, maintains the highest standards of excellence, and offers a full and complete array of care modalities.

- The right to healing even when there is no cure.

- The right to be whole.[25]

Change is Coming

Traditionally, the conventional medical community has been suspicious of Ayurveda, Traditional Chinese Medicine, medicinal herbs, hydrotherapy, vitamin supplementation, meditation and numerous other modalities associated with complementary and alternative medicine, many of which are found in spas worldwide. But even the most entrenched attitudes are susceptible to change.

By the end of the first decade of the 21st century, three significant factors had converged to signal a potential shift from a reactive to more proactive approach in medical care:

- The efforts of many enlightened members of the medical community over the past decades that have heightened the awareness of a more personal and constructive approach to individual wellness and a more integrative approach to medicine;

- A growing body of evidence-based research from around the world that is capturing the attention of the conventional medical community;

- The exigencies of spiraling health care costs along with the coming of (retirement) age of the first of the Baby Boomers in 2011.

Doctors Making a Difference

Over the years, a critical mass of individual doctors and institutions has been quietly but inexorably conducting studies and implementing innovative programs throughout North America.

For example, at the government level, the U.S. National Institutes of Health have undertaken numerous studies and initiatives relating to complementary and alternative medicine (CAM) through the National Center for Complementary and Alternative Medicine and the Office of Dietary Supplements.

And within academia, The Bravewell Collaborative and the Consortium of Academic Health Centers for Integrative Medicine (more than 50 medical centers from the US and Canada, including Harvard Medical School, Yale University, Mayo Clinic, Johns Hopkins University and Duke University), support and mentor academic leaders, faculty and students to advance integrative healthcare curricula, research and clinical care.[26]

The individual doctors below represent medical doctors that I have personally had the privilege of experiencing over the past two decades. They represent only a few of the pioneers in complementary and integrative medicine that have been responsible for heightening awareness and legitimizing these concepts both within the conventional medical community and the general public:

- *Dr. Mehmet Oz, MD, FACS,* vice-chair and professor of Surgery at Columbia University College of Physician's and Surgeons and Medical Director, Integrative Medicine Program at NY Presbyterian Hospital, Columbia University Medical Center, New York, and well-known host of The Dr. Oz Show, promotes a medical evidence-based approach to preventive health care and is seen by millions of viewers daily.

- *Dr. Brent Bauer, MD, FACS,* Director of the Department of Internal Medicine's Complementary and Integrative Medicine Program at Mayo Clinic, Rochester, MN for the last 20 years has focused on the scientific evaluation CAM therapies at this prestigious health center.

- *Dr. Dean Ornish, MD,* with his not-for-profit Preventive Medicine Research Institute, has led the way in cardiac rehabilitation through his four pillars of health: Nutrition, Exercise, Stress Management and Spirituality supported by evidence-based research conducted by his Institute and elsewhere.

- *Dr. Kenneth Cooper, MD, MPH,* the "Father of Aerobics" at his Cooper Institute has been collecting scientific data on physical fitness, physical activity and health for over 30 years and is recognized as a leader and educator in the areas of preventive medicine and wellness through diet, exercise and emotional/mental balance.

- *Dr. Andrew Weil, MD,* perhaps one of the most famous doctors in the field of Complementary and Integrative Medicine, founder and director of the Program in Integrative Medicine (PIM) at the University of Arizona in Tucson, often controversial for his views on alternative medicine particularly within the mainstream medical community, yet instrumental in promoting complementary medicine, has had an immensely positive impact on its acceptability and popularity within the general public.

- *Dr. Kenneth Pelletier, PhD, MD, HC,* Director, Corporate Health Improvement Program and clinical professor of Medicine at both the University of Arizona School of Medicine and the University of

Maryland School of Medicine; clinical professor of Medicine and psychiatry, University of California School of Medicine in San Francisco (UCSF) and president of the American Health Association, is an authority and recognized leader in the fields of alternative and integrative medicine.

There are, of course, many other doctors and physicians from hospitals, universities, medical centers and medical schools on an international scale without whose contributions, as a society, we might not have arrived at this point – poised to embrace a more integrated medical system with a greater emphasis on prevention.

Dr. Brent Bauer, MD, FACS, Director of the Complementary and Integrative Medicine Program at the Mayo Clinic, Rochester, MN:

"The medical community is increasingly recognizing the profound effects that stress has on patients. With this recognition comes a growing acceptance of therapies geared to minimizing the effects of stress – e.g. meditation, massage, guided imagery, etc. This reflects a unique opportunity for medicine and spa to work more closely together to optimize patient health and wellness."

Evidence-based Medical Research

The body of research in the area of complementary and alternative medicine (CAM) has grown dramatically (more than 16,000 studies, up from 9,861 in 2006). In these clinical studies, a host of conditions including stress, cancer, blood pressure, insomnia and arthritis have been proven to be significantly alleviated by modalities such as massage, meditation, yoga, acupuncture and nutrition (please keep in mind that these modalities are complementary in that they do not necessarily replace the medical treatments, rather alleviate symptoms, often helping to hasten the healing process).

In light of this growing body of evidence, many mainstream doctors, hospitals and medical centers are beginning to look for ways to integrate CAM into their own practices and organizations.

This vast body of data needs to be accumulated, collated and aggregated. One data base, the Natural Standard organization comprised of healthcare providers and researchers, gathers and evaluates data from around the world and makes it available on a subscription basis to healthcare professionals, insurers, manufacturers, retailers and the consumer. This evidence-based, peer-reviewed, consensus-driven, high quality information is intended to provide all stakeholders in the area of Health and Wellness with the tools for making informed decisions regarding complementary and alternative therapies.

In addition to Natural Standard, the Cochrane Collaborative, PubMed.gov and the Trip Database are the other primary relevant, evidence-based medicine databases accessed by the medical community.

And spas? Although they offer many of the modalities that have been scientifically studied, for the most part they have not connected the dots in order to use this available body of research in promoting their businesses. Awareness of these studies, as well as understanding how to adapt the information they provide, will change thanks to an initiative proposed by Dr. Kenneth Pelletier at the 2010 Global Spa Summit in Istanbul, Turkey and vigorously supported and promoted by spa industry leader Susie Ellis of SpaFinder Inc. and others (the Global Spa Summit is "an international organization that brings together leaders and visionaries to positively impact and shape the future of the global spa and wellness industry" and has been meeting in different countries around the world since 2006).

As a result of this event, several well-known medical doctors and spa industry professionals formed a commission to further develop and implement the proposed initiative, christening it "SpaEvidence, The Science Behind Wellness Therapies."

For each of the 21 wellness categories, there is an overview of the modality; a spotlight per category of five or six studies from around the world; completed research from each of the four databases listed above and finally studies currently in progress at ClinicalTrials.gov and the World Health Organization.

This ground-breaking site, www.spaevidence.com, enables spas and consumers like you to share and profit from the valuable information contained in these studies. Specifically, as a consumer, this research provides you with a little more knowledge and hopefully a better understanding from a scientific point of view of the many benefits of the wellness therapies that you find in your spa. It's easy to navigate and once you get started digging, like eating popcorn, it's hard to stop.

If you already are a classical E-patient[27] – one who uses the internet to gather data from many different sites to use in evaluating the quality of your family's and your own medical care, both preventive and clinical – this site will be of special interest. Whether you use it to encourage your physician to employ a more integrative approach to your own personal health care is up to you.

An inspiring example of the possibilities that evidence-based research can open up for all types of spas through forming partnerships with the medical community is the Inspiritas Spa at the START Center for Cancer Care in San Antonio, Texas. Opened in late 2010, cancer patients along with their families, friends and caregivers can find manipulative therapies, such as massage; energy therapies, like reiki; biological therapies, which include nutrition-related treatments; mind/body intervention, including psychotherapy, guided imagery and meditation; and whole medical systems, such as acupuncture in a true spa setting. As noted, all of these modalities are supported by evidence-based research and are provided to reduce the patient's stress and increase his or her sense of wellbeing. In turn, these modalities are able to help his or her immune system operate more efficiently and even support the healing process.

Baby Boomers Influence Health Care

Baby Boomers, one of the most influential demographic groups in history (75.8 million of them born between 1946 and 1964), were raised in the post WWII era and defined by prosperity, children in the spotlight, television, suburbia, assassinations, Vietnam, civil rights, the Cold War, women's liberation and the space race.

Although conventional medicine was their primary health care source, they made exercise and aerobics popular in the 60's and 70's and segued into spa and wellness by the 90's, with many of them subsequently joining movements like the $290 billion L.O.H.A.S. (Lifestyles of Health and Sustainability) that embraces sustainability and wellness.

Today, with skyrocketing health care costs, exacerbated by the specter of huge medical bills eating up their retirement incomes as the first of them hit the age of 65 in 2011, a good number of Boomers (followed by Gen-Xer's and Yer's) are seeking alternatives to a medical and health care system that focuses primarily on intervention and cure rather than prevention. Look for Boomers as a whole to continue to exert their considerable influence and for the health care system, including Medicare, to respond accordingly.

A Tip of the Hat to Two Great Motivators in My Life

Two individuals, one very old-fashioned and one very modern, heavily influenced my conviction that we are personally responsible for staying as healthy as we possibly can. They either were or are medical doctors whose dedication to their profession has continued to inspire and motivate their patients and those with whom they've interacted.

The Old Guard

The first, my grandfather, Dr. Hugh B. Fate, MD, decided to pursue a medical degree after having reached the position of High School principal in eastern Washington State. He packed up his wife and three kids and moved to Los Angeles, receiving his MD at Los Angeles' Loma Linda University. He went on to become a country doctor in Eastern Oregon during the 1930's and 40's, and in the 50's established a thriving practice in Fairbanks, Alaska as an eye specialist (EENT). He also was one of Alaska's flying bush doctors, providing medical care in remote locations for whites and native Indians alike throughout this vast state.

Dr. Fate was a big man with a totally bald pate who sported a beret, a hearty, booming "har, har, har" laugh and political views that put him somewhere to the right of Attila the Hun. He loved horse racing and raised and trained racehorses at various junctures in his life, always hoping that "this one is the one."

I remember many things about this larger-than-life man, but what stands out in my mind most clearly was his absolute, and oft-stated, conviction that "the healing process consists of 25% medicine and 75% the relationship between doctor and patient." He said this even though he was witness, over the better part of the 20th century, to the many (often seemingly miraculous) advances in every aspect of health care, making use of them just as every other doctor does who lives by the Hippocratic Oath.

He did not in any way gainsay the efficacy of conventional medicine. But since the local pharmacy back then looked vastly different from ours today and when faced with many, if not most, of the same ailments suffered by today's patients, he had to be innovative in his approach. Depending on the financial wherewithal of his patients who often didn't have sufficient financial resources (as an old-fashioned country doctor, he accepted payment in whatever form possible – dollars, chickens, produce and services), he had to find ways to provide these people the medical care and treatments he felt they deserved.

My grandfather realized that a simple conversation involving listening carefully, perceptively and respectfully to his patient and then offering a simple course of action or even a kind word could often be as effective as a prescription for a medication.

As part of his "treatment arsenal," he practiced and understood the mind-body relationship long before the term was coined and he preached this credo up to his death in 1978.

The New Order

The second MD to whom I'd like to tip my hat is Dr. Pamela Peeke, MD, MPH, FACP, who served as medical advisor to the International Spa Association Board of Directors during the years that I was a member of that board. Dr. Pam is one of the few physicians (unfortunately still a minority) with advanced training in the field of nutrition and is equally able in the areas of metabolism, stress and fitness. She was the first senior research fellow at the National Institutes of Health Office of Alternative Medicine where she helped establish the scientific foundation for the research and development of investigations involving nutrition and fitness. Her national bestsellers, *Fight Fat After Forty,* followed by *Body for Life for Women* and her newest, *Fit to Live,* have provided millions of women (and men) a better understanding of the relationship between stress and the size of their waistlines.

She is also one of the wittiest, most energetic women I have ever met. When she lasers you with a look from her bright, blue eyes and makes a point, you know you'd better sit up and take notice. She is a born leader who inspires countless women through her commitment to "walking the talk" and is a sought after expert for a variety of talk shows, host of her own TV show, a Pew

Foundation Scholar in Nutrition and Metabolism and Assistant Professor of Medicine at the University of Maryland. Frankly, her bio wears me out![28]

As a dedicated advisor to the ISPA board in the 90's, she continually searched for ways to bring together allopathic medicine and the different modalities that were then termed alternative, as well as to give credibility to the holistic mind, body, spirit approach of Spa. Through her work at the NIH, she was in contact with the few universities, private clinics or medical institutions at the time that were conducting research into these alternative modalities, such as Harvard Medical School, Dr. Andrew Weil, Dr. Larry Dossey, Deepak Chopra, Dr. Kenneth Cooper, Dr. Kenneth Pelletier and others.

Today, Dr. Pamela Peeke is an expert in the newly emerging field of gender specific health and medicine, emphasizing the strengths and vulnerabilities of both genders as they practice healthy lifestyles. She is the Medical Director of the National Women's Health Resource Center, in addition to being a member of Oprah Winfrey's "O Team" of nationally recognized experts in women's health and a tireless advocate for the benefits of integrative medicine.

Both my grandfather and Dr. Peeke represent the future of medicine – a balanced, integrated, respectful and holistic approach to a patient's total wellbeing through the integration of a variety of wellness modalities and conventional medical therapies.

The Travelling Spa Goer

Today's spa consumer is more mobile than ever, traveling for business or pleasure to far away destinations all over the globe. The concept of wellness tourism has evolved from the choices many consumers are making to incorporate aspects of wellness into their activities once at their chosen destinations.

The information below is a synopsis of a 2011 Global Spa Summit report that I have included because, in the coming years, your travel choices and destination activities in terms of spas and wellness will be more focused and made easier thanks to the efforts of this remarkable group.

In 2010 the Global Spa Summit's report, *Spas and the Global Wellness Market: Synergies and Opportunities*, had estimated the Wellness Tourism sector globally at US$106B compared with Medical Tourism at US$50B showing how robust the wellness tourism sector already is compared with medical tourism and providing impetus for further study.[29]

The Global Spa Summit 2011 focused on spas and wellness with the presentation of a ground-breaking research report entitled *Wellness Tourism and Medical Tourism: Where Do Spas Fit?* that covers the emergence of medical tourism and wellness tourism around the world.

The relatively new wellness tourism and medical tourism sectors are still considered niche markets by most nations, presenting challenges for growth on a global scale. The underlying, fundamental problem has been the lack of coherent definitions of the terms wellness tourism and medical tourism.

The report proposed that the spa industry adopt the following definitions in order to better work together with these industries:

Medical tourism involves people who travel to a different place to receive treatment for a disease, an ailment, or a condition, or to undergo a cosmetic procedure, and who are seeking a lower cost of care, higher quality of care, better access to care or different care than what they could receive at home.

Medical tourist: Generally ill or seeking cosmetic or dental surgical procedures or enhancements.

Wellness tourism involves people who travel to a different place to proactively pursue activities that maintain or enhance their personal health and wellbeing, and who are seeking unique, authentic or location-based experiences/therapies not available at home.

Wellness tourist. Generally seeking integrated wellness and prevention approaches to improve their health/quality of life.

Twelve countries were selected as case studies based on their representative geographic location and past and current efforts in the areas of wellness and medical tourism, with Canada representing North America.

It was determined that spas should concentrate initially on growing their presence in the wellness tourism sector, since spas worldwide have played a significant part in wellness tourism in the past due to their obvious wellness focus.

My Conclusions?

As wellness tourism matures, you will be given a wider, more coherent array of options and far more definitive information as you make your wellness travel choices based on the type of spa experience you seek, eg. holistic or longevity retreats and cruises; ashrams; boot camps; nutrition and weight loss/detox retreats; active retreats with hiking, golf, tennis, water sports, etc. and/or eco retreats with a wellness focus.

Though only the beginning, the Global Spa Summit initiatives are a significant step in pointing the way for spas to re-evaluate their programs and step into the wellness arena.

And the Future?

As spas and the health care community move ever closer, as a consumer you can look for and/or promote:

- More and more evidence-based research that supports the benefits of massage, yoga, nutrition, exercise, meditation, acupuncture and other modalities making them increasingly accepted as part of your doctor's arsenal of treatments along with conventional drugs and therapies.

- Mainstream spas moving towards wellness as they stress the therapeutic, indigenous aspects of their treatments, as well as increasingly incorporating programs in healthy aging, lifestyle coaching, nutritional counselling, etc., in order to actively promote the health and wellbeing of their guests.

- A wider acceptance and integration of spa therapies such as massage and hydrotherapy into the programs of hospitals and medical centers.

- Increasing coverage by HMO's and Medicare of programs such as the Ornish Program for Reversing Heart Disease that focus on lifestyle changes such as diet, exercise, stress management and emotional and spiritual health.

On A Personal Note

A lifetime of exposure to the concept of taking personal responsibility for the health of myself and my family has resulted in "treating" all of us with simple home remedies, good food and an avoidance of doctor's offices except for emergencies and real illness — though not in an irrational or dogmatic way, by any stretch of the imagination. We've seen our fair share of emergency rooms and an annual physical is part of our routines, but so are vitamins, meditation, long walks, Pilates and visits to the spa enabling us to remain healthy and active human beings.

I want to encourage you to at least investigate a more integrative approach to your health — including diet and exercise, attention to your spiritual self and looking for alternatives to pharmaceuticals to keep you well — along with regular visits to your doctor and following his or her medical advice and/or courses of treatment. The one does not preclude the other.

Fortunately, I have learned that spas are an equally vital component of my health equation, allowing me the time and giving me the space to breathe, heal and find compassionate care in our often frenetic world. Make spas part of yours. For your health!

Chapter 14 Eat to Live and Move to Eat

Spas and wellness are about living in balance through rejuvenating treatments, proper diet, restful sleep, adequate exercise, meditation and appropriate lifestyle choices. Consequently, no book about the value of spas and spa-going would be complete without the mention of fitness and nutrition. And though not every spa features them, nutrition and fitness nevertheless round out the spa picture.

Spas and Nutrition

The evolution of modern Spa Cuisine had its genesis seventy years ago at Rancho La Puerta, North America's seminal spa. Edward and Deborah Szekely's insistence on fresh vegetables and fruits, legumes, whole grains and an ovo-lactarian diet, that has undergone only moderate changes over the years, set the stage for the fat farms of the 50's, 60's, 70's and 80's where (predominantly well-heeled) women would pay big bucks for minimally caloric dishes, often devoid of taste, in order to lose weight.

In the late 80's and early 90's, the notion that food could look and taste good, be nutritious and contribute to weight loss caused Spa Food to begin its metamorphosis to Spa Cuisine. At the same time that scientific evidence for the nutritional value of food began to mount, "clean" food production moved out of the spa and into those restaurants whose creative chefs had been experimenting with herbs, spices and innovative combinations of ingredients, taking their cues from often-exotic kitchens from around the world. This in turn influenced many spa chefs to retool their menus to make them more tasty and flavorful, realizing that their patrons' palates had become a good deal more sophisticated over the years.

In the spa, nutritionists replaced dieticians, and pioneers like Cheryl Hartsough, Sheila Cluff and Edward Safdie actively promoted this new form of food preparation. Sauces were no longer taboo – rather they were made without a heavy emphasis on butter and cream, using herbs and spices and low fat/low sodium stocks and broths to enhance them. Patrons were offered a wider variety of choices as a broad range of organically grown salads, vegetables and fruits became available. And as time progressed, free range chicken, fish and whole eggs found their way back onto spa menus, while even wine in moderation became acceptable at some spas.

Today, delicious and delectable have become legitimate descriptions of our modern Spa Cuisine. Chefs in a number of leading hotel and resort spas worldwide are recognized by foodies as culinary stars and celebrity chefs from around the world are invited to spas to share their culinary prowess.

Chef Laurie Ericson, acclaimed wellness chef and culinary educator with a pedigree that reads like a "Who's Who" of spas, prefers to refer to spa cuisine simply as healthy eating.

She notes that spa chefs now focus on organic, locally grown and sustainable foods – foods that have become functional with a focus on maximizing nutritional value. On their menus look for sustainably harvested fish, free range poultry and eggs, grass-fed beef and organic dairy products.

What else are they doing? They know that the type of fat is more important than the amount of fat in a healthful diet. Unsaturated fats like olive, soybean, canola and nut oils, and especially the Omega 3 fats found in fish, walnuts, canola oil, and soybean oil, appear on menus formerly boasting about their "low fat" content. Refined grains and sugar have yielded to whole grain breads, pastas and a variety of rice. Veggies are served roasted for their flavour and retention of their natural goodness, while a panoply of herbs and spices are used to intensify flavour and taste. Vegetables and fruits known for their anti-oxidant values (primarily beta-carotene, vitamin C and vitamin E that help fight the cellular damage that leads to aging) are the colourful ones: yellow, green, purple, blue, red and orange.

Chefs have become educators with a mission, striving to awaken the palates of their spa guests and give them the tools and information to continue a healthier lifestyle at home – exemplified by Chef Laurie during her stints as demonstration chef at Canyon Ranch Resort in the Berkshires and wellness chef at The Cloisters in Sea Island, GA. She emphasizes, "Healthy food doesn't mean that it doesn't taste good."

Chef Laurie's Delicious and Delectable Fine Spa Cuisine

"Here is my Dream Dinner - of course the vegetables are organic and the fish wild and fresh."

Roasted Baby Beet Salad with Arugula and Walnut Crusted Goat Cheese, Aged Balsamic and Extra Virgin Olive Oil

225 calories 3 grams fat

~

Vegetable Consommé with Julienne Asian Vegetables, Fresh Ginger and Cilantro

160 calories .5 grams fat

~

Wasabi Pea-crusted Wild Salmon with Black Sticky Rice and Sautéed Rainbow Chard

358 calories 7 grams fat

~

Lime Pots de Crème with Fresh Blueberries (Dairy Free)

157 calories 5 grams fat

Chef Laurie Erickson,
author of *Chef by Step®*
The World's Easiest Cookbook

Helping people understand that it is a simple step-by-step commitment to changing their eating patterns is her goal. She suggests choosing ten things that you want to change and then making those changes one at a time rather than trying to do them all at once – perhaps not a completely novel suggestion, but certainly a compelling one.

Spa cuisine `a la Chef Laurie is the perfect vehicle for learning more about eating for a healthy lifestyle.

Weight Loss Spas

Let's call it weight management, shall we? Whether destination spas, boot camps or even some resort spas, they offer some type of weight management program that can be customized to suit your particular needs. There are also specialty spas that exclusively target weight loss with calorie-controlled menus and specific programming. They combine nutritious food with vigorous exercise programs, including hiking, yoga, Pilates and fitness training, along with classes in cooking and nutrition (as well as a variety of other creative and educational workshops and classes) in order to provide tools and the motivation for you to continue your healthier lifestyle at home.

Many health spas that offer these programs, like Rancho La Puerta, Canyon Ranch, Green Mountain Spa, Miraval, Mii Amo and others, are located in breathtaking settings that nurture the spirit and allow you to focus solely on meeting your goals and making the most of your spa week. Some of these spas also offer detox and/or cleansing programs that help your body eliminate the toxins that have accumulated due to our often less than healthy lifestyles. A few spas, especially amongst destination spas, offer counselling from qualified, on-staff medical professionals to further ensure the safety and effectiveness of their programs.

It doesn't matter whether you want to lose a little or a lot of weight, spas can provide the perfect environment for you to optimize your desired outcome.

Nutrition Today

Spa savvy, educated consumers have been nutritionally aware for many years, looking at not only the caloric content of their food, but also its sodium, fat and carbohydrate content. This awareness has begun to gain traction in the general public through the quantity of useful, well-researched, evidence-based information available on the web and television. Dr. Mehmud Oz and chefs like Britain's Jamie Oliver or Nathan Lyon of the Food Network are at the forefront of educating their viewing audiences about healthy foods and food preparation (found, not coincidentally, in spas), in addition to numerous websites like Dr. Weil's Weekly Bulletin.

As a sidebar: the use of nutritional supplementation has continued to increase, with a growing number of people who lead a healthy lifestyle making dietary supplements part of their daily regimen.

Nevertheless, even with all the strides being made with regards to consumer awareness, information and education in the areas of obesity and nutrition, effecting a change and a shift in consumer attitudes towards a healthier lifestyle remains an enormous challenge.

 The Junk Food Plague

The great dichotomy between the horrendous consumption of unhealthy, fast (junk) food and the increasing popularity and availability of organic and nutritionally sound foods continues to widen and confound.

Junk Foods and Obesity

The sociological reasons for the rise in obesity in North America are many and varied, with studies, commissions, programs and legislation conducted over the past few years aimed at explaining and dealing with the phenomenon, especially amongst children and youth. Yet one in three persons in the United States and one in four in Canada are clinically obese.

Alarmingly, a study representative of all Americans, based on patterns found in the National Health and Nutrition Examination Surveys (NHANES) from 1988 to 2008, projects that by 2020, 83% of men and 72% of women will be overweight or obese if present trends continue.

The socio-economic implications for an increasingly obese society are staggering – in 2008 reaching around $US147 billion.[30] Obesity can lead to more than 20 chronic diseases, including Type 2 diabetes, coronary heart disease, osteoarthritis and high blood pressure, resulting in decreased productivity and personal loss of income through restricted activity, absenteeism and sick days.

Obesity-related diseases already have a substantial impact on the health care system that will continue to grow as the population ages.

The "Surgeon General's Vision for a Healthy and Fit Nation" released in 2010 in the US and the Public Health Agency of Canada's 2011 white paper "Obesity in Canada" speak directly to the effects of obesity and overweight in the immediate and long-terms in both North American populations. They emphasize the need for a comprehensive approach that engages both the public and private sectors in homes, schools, daycares, work places and at the communal level.

But what of our youth in the short term? Unfortunately, nutrition education in schools hasn't been able to compete with the overwhelming number of ads for candy, sodas, snacks and junk food bombarding kids on a daily basis. And the many technological innovations – games, phones, and a plethora of products that keep kids on sofas and inactive – only exacerbate the problem. When you add to that the decrease in physical education in so many schools due to lack of funding and the fact that fast foods are cheaper for families living at the subsistence and/or poverty level, you have many of the problems we face today.

So, to what extent all the initiatives aimed at a healthier population can be effective depends on daycare operators, school lunchrooms and us as parents getting behind the efforts of organizations, individuals and governments to combat this growing problem.

The Opportunity for Spas

The opportunity for spas to offer more than wellness and pampering for a person's "outside" has never been greater. Adding nutritional counselling to spa treatment menus and reintroducing fitness programming, either in the spa or in partnership with local fitness establishments, can have a significant impact on the attitudes and actions of a spa's guests.

As spas consciously move into the wellness arena, there is an opportunity for them to find ways to incorporate nutrition education in their community outreach programs - truly valuable for both spas and the general public. The Canyon Ranch Institute, for example, has proven that spas can make a difference (even though not every spa has Canyon Ranch's resources) no matter how small the contribution.

It is especially encouraging that in 2010, four million teens went to spas to learn about stress management and nutrition, demonstrating that there is a willingness amongst at least some of today's youth to choose healthy eating over the convenience and appeal that junk foods have to a kid's palate.

Fit for Life

From the earliest days of the modern spa era, fitness has played an integral part in spa programming. Up through the early 90's, as destination spas were still in the ascendency in terms of defining the spa experience, there was no question that movement and exercise were as necessary to a well-rounded spa program as healthy food. And as resort/hotel spas entered the spa scene, they emulated their destination counterparts, including a fitness component in their facilities, as well.

However, that practice began to decline throughout the past decade so that by 2010 only a little over 60% of resort/hotel spas included fitness of some kind.[31] The same study showed that an average of one in ten spas (54% of resort/hotels spas, but only 7% of day spas) offered actual fitness or sports services ranging from cardio training to yoga and Pilates to personal training.

 ## Ruth Stricker - A Perfect Example

Back in the late 70's and early 80's, the fitness movement had already become a household word throughout North America. Young Ruth Stricker, another remarkable visionary, was part of this movement as a fitness instructor, first in Massachusetts and later in Minnesota, with a keen interest in the relationship between mind and body. She realized early on that wellness was more than strong muscles and a toned body; it involved caring for the whole person, listening, encouraging, supporting them mentally and emotionally as well as physically.

But sometimes, bad things happen to good people and Ruth developed systemic Lupus, a chronic and debilitating autoimmune disorder, at the tender age of forty. Characteristically, she decided that this disease would not rule her life and came to terms with her illness in a positive and ultimately more constructive way.

She founded The Marsh in Minnetonka, Minnesota, in 1985 as A Center for Balance and Fitness, based on years of study of Eastern philosophy, fitness and wholistic medicine. With the backing of Bruce Dayton, who became her husband three years later, she built a 67,000 sq. ft. center that incorporated a place for people from all walks of life to come for professional care and guidance for a healthier lifestyle. The Marsh offers a communal environment that integrates exercise, health and nutritional education, therapeutic treatments (body work), a caring staff and a variety of programs focusing on everything from weight loss to stress relief. Interestingly, her focus has stayed constant and steady and the programs today mirror those of 26 years ago.

The exercise programs at The Marsh, with their mindful and cognitive approach, attracted the attention of the medical community in Minnesota and local medical professionals began recommending her classes to their patients for a more balanced approach to dealing with their illnesses. Today, the Mayo Clinic regularly sends patients to The Marsh to adjust and recuperate from surgeries.

The Marsh features a fitness centre, Pilates studio, a mental gym, a meditation tower, a full service spa, a physical therapy clinic, restaurants, overnight guest rooms, a retail shop and meeting and event spaces along with a professional staff of cardiologist, exercise physiologist, dietitian, acupuncturist and exercise specialists.

Ruth Stricker has remained deeply involved in her community – locally and globally – throughout her life and in recognition of her lifetime contribution in the field of spa was awarded the 2004 Alex Szekely Humanitarian Award from the International Spa and Fitness Association, in addition to the many other national and international honours and awards she has garnered. She continues to give generously of herself and her resources and is highly revered within the spa industry for her passionate belief in the integration of medicine and wellness.

Of the resort/hotel spas that include fitness areas, many are extensive and often include paid memberships for locals. More often than not, as a hotel guest, for a day use fee you can use the spa's exercise and water facilities (pool, sauna, steam room, etc.) without actually using the spa, per se. These spas also tend to offer mind/body activities, such as tai chi, yoga, Pilates and meditation classes, bringing the notion of "mindfulness" into the fitness equation and emphasizing the Mind, Body and Spirit aspects of spa. As previously noted, as spas of all types adopt a more wellness-focused approach, they will hopefully reintroduce fitness back into their programming.

Over the past few years, wellness and this mindful approach to fitness has also found its way into the health and fitness clubs of North America. Pilates, Yoga and personal training have become increasingly popular, giving rise to the club spa. Most club spas can be found in urban areas and were initially offshoots of the fitness clubs in which they're located. Club spas that combine fitness activities and spa services and treatments now make up 2.8% of the total number of spas in the United States.

Fitness Outside the Spa

The health and fitness industry is here to stay! A blinding flash of the obvious? Perhaps so, but with the obesity epidemic continuing unabated, it does make you wonder. Interestingly, according to the IDEA Health and Fitness Association, as of 2010, more than 70% of adult women and 60% of adult men got no regular exercise and nearly half of young people aged 12-21 did not participate in any sort of vigorous physical activity, the consequences of which present a huge challenge for the public and private sectors (see Junk Food Plague above).

In 2010, IDEA launched its Inspire the World to Fitness®, a broad-based initiative to utilize the fitness industry as a powerful and effective force to combat obesity. They argue that the industry has evolved more thorough, increased training knowledge and more sophisticated, specialized equipment, allowing it to become more responsive to the variety of fitness levels and abilities of its clientele and making it more attractive to a broader range of individuals. In order to combat a "fatter" and "sicker" world they have pledged their membership to make a difference.

What's in Store

Back in the spa, perhaps the advent of intuitive technology, easily customized to hold the interest and spark the imagination of the user, can help reincorporate fitness into the spa scene. As the consumer integrates all of his or her activities into a cohesive wellness plan through Network Fitness (see below), he or she might begin to demand the one-stop convenience, complemented by the calmer atmosphere that a spa can provide.

 ## Network Fitness

Couch potato alert! Things are changing thanks to one of the same reasons that keeps people glued to their seats – technology. The intriguing and innovative advances in intuitive consoles over the past few years is changing the way fitness equipment can be customized to suit the client.

For fitness professionals, the question has always been how to quantify the amount and effectiveness of their clients' movements, especially when the individual isn't in the spa or fitness centre, resulting in the proliferation of personal tracking devices like pedometers. Wi-Fi provided the answer and has changed everything.

Enter network fitness, enabling you to virtually track your every movement, store that information in the Cloud and access it from any point on the globe. Spearheaded by the fitness equipment company, Precor, an acknowledged market leader with consistently cutting-edge technology, network fitness is now a reality.

The implications of network fitness are enormous. For example, through personal devices, each and every movement you make can be quantified and stored. Let's assume that your doctor has determined that you should follow a daily exercise regimen for a specific ailment or condition. Up until now, it wasn't possible to effectively track your movements – especially to determine the amount of energy used in activities like parking your car on the other side of the parking lot or taking three flights of stairs rather than the elevator – outside of "official" time working out in a fitness club or in specific activities like walking for 20 minutes, etc. Now, through the Network, your physician will be able to monitor and evaluate your program and tweak it to maximize your fitness outcome. Imagine the possibilities!

These devices can be synched with machines and related equipment found in fitness clubs and spas and are software driven, with you performing the same sweeping motions you do with your phones and other devices on touch screens similar to ATM's and airport check-in terminals. The full Wi-Fi gamut allows you to tailor your fitness programs, and features docking stations for IPods, a wide variety of TV and VOD programs and connectivity with other equipment.

Since equipment can be programmed and updated without needing replacement, it makes the concept of network fitness highly attractive and economical to spa and fitness facilities' owners and operators. In turn, wouldn't you find a visit to their facilities more compelling, fun and desirable?

Nutrition and fitness are some of the keys to solving many of the problems besetting our society, globally, arising from health or medically-related causes for young and old alike. The efforts of dedicated spa enthusiasts and spa professionals, in tandem with public and private initiatives, have the potential to help stem the tide by heightening awareness, providing education and motivating every person who walks in their doors – a truly golden opportunity.

Chapter 15 How It Really All Began

There have always been rare individuals who have had a vision coupled with the passion and staying power to realize their dreams. Perhaps it's because they aren't in it for the fame and glory, but out of a deep-seated conviction that what they do has value – not only personally, but also for society in general.

Think of Steve Jobs tinkering away with his friends in his garage knowing that developing a computer for personal use was not only possible, but could be made affordable for the average guy. Consider the scientist in a laboratory plugging away day after day after day in search of a cure for cancer. Or all those who put in hours of effort, throwing in whatever cash they can scrape together to make their visions reality and who then possess the power to inspire everyone around them to follow their vision with the same fire and passion.

This chapter is devoted to two incredible women who have helped shape the spa industry and have had an extraordinary influence in making Spa a household word. Each has pursued her vision of Spa from her own perspective and the contributions of each to the modern spa and wellness movement are invaluable.

Both have inspired me, personally, through their ongoing dedication and perseverance to evolving the conviction that Spa is about a person's overall health and wellness, with pampering merely a side benefit of the overall spa experience.

Deborah Szekely – The Ultimate Spa Icon

The evolution of the spa as we know it today had its roots in Tecate, Mexico back in 1940. The acclaimed doyenne of the spa industry, Deborah Szekely, then 17 years old, followed her new husband, Professor Edmund Szekely, a renaissance man who believed in drawing from ancient cultures, as well as the latest in philosophy, science and medicine, to Tecate where they opened the doors of North America's seminal destination spa. Today a sprawling complex of casitas, lush gardens and swimming pools on 3,000 acres at the foot of the magical, chaparral-covered Mount Kuchumaa, Rancho La Puerta started as a one-room adobe hut sitting in the middle of a vineyard, where guests were expected to pitch in and help alongside workers drawn from the surrounding Mexican countryside.

They lived by the Professor's essential philosophy:

"To survive in this increasingly artificial world, mankind must reprise old ways of eating nutritiously and moving naturally, and in so doing establish new ways of achieving balance and realizing one's entire potential. So can we lead a useful, long, healthful life!"

From the beginning, Rancho La Puerta used organic farming methods for an abundant supply of fruits and vegetables. Goats were there to produce milk and cheese. Fresh air, simple "spa" food and an environment that encouraged meditation and contemplation drew guests that participated in nearly every aspect of the community's day-to-day life. Simplicity was the order of the day.

Word spread about the Rancho through their informative and educational monthly bulletins and the prolific works of the Professor who gave daily lectures and experimented with theories old and new, such as the use of Dr. Sebastian Kneipp's hydrotherapy techniques; yoga; solar energy and employing herbs and vitamins for optimal health, amongst other pursuits. Many of the ground-breaking concepts developed by him at that time have been validated by research today.

But Deborah soon realized that guests were looking for more in the way of physical activity and other diversions, so she looked for ways to make old-fashioned calisthenics more enjoyable. Music was the answer and eventually Deborah began hiring instructors with backgrounds in modern dance, along with others with fitness degrees, in order to offer a program that encompassed a variety of disciplines from exercising to jazz music to hatha yoga. Today, Rancho La Puerta offers more than 75 different mind, body and spirit classes from a variety of different disciplines that change weekly depending on the guest lecturers and instructors in attendance.

Back in the 50's, however, many guests demanded a more sophisticated and luxurious atmosphere in which to learn about and experience the Szekely philosophy of health, fitness and nutrition – leading to the opening of the Golden Door in Escondido, California in 1958. It drew on the experience and knowledge gleaned from Rancho La Puerta, but in a very exclusive and luxurious way, basing its ambience and design on the ancient Honjin inns of Japan.

Deborah is the acknowledged co-founder of the modern day fitness movement that paved the way for other health spas that were to feature weight-loss, beauty and physical fitness. These became known as "fat farms," catering to the rich and famous and influencing the perceptions of a generation of individuals for whom the word Spa would become synonymous with pampering and fluff. But for the hundreds of thousands of guests of Rancho La Puerta and the Golden Door, who have fallen under their spell and experienced life-altering moments at these superb spas, Deborah's philosophy has given them the inspiration and motivation to embrace all that these spas epitomize with enthusiasm.

The most impressive fact is that Rancho La Puerta has remained true to Deborah's vision to this day. As you meander along the interconnecting brick paths, inhaling the fragrant and uplifting air, you encounter a burbling fountain here or the jewelled waters of a pool there, drawing you on to explore and appreciate the serenity and beauty of your surroundings. Yet it's totally unpretentious, even understated, and as comfortable as an old shoe – evident in the faces of the guests sporting the Rancho's trademark black shoulder totes and personalized water bottles who nod smilingly as you pass by. Even the gardeners are friendly, proud of the work they do and the magic they create. An abundance of trees and cacti of every description shelters walkers from the heat of the sun, while rounded bronze sculptures dotting the grounds celebrate Woman in her various attitudes. You are struck by the fact that every last detail has been organically woven into a sublime whole over the past 70 years.

The appetizing, gourmet food is no "in your face" vegan fare, just deliciously satisfying and elegantly presented. A visit to The Rancho's organic farm, Rancho Tres Estrellas and its splendid demo kitchen where guests come to learn the secrets to healthy and nutritious cuisine, often from a roster of talented guest chefs, is a sensory delight. Fragrant herbs, larger than life vegetables and flowers grow in colourful profusion on the six acres of Tres Estrellas under the watchful eye of head gardener, Salvador Tinajero. A 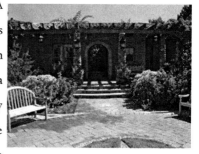 magnificent smile and earth-stained hands are the hallmark of this charismatic man who has been with Rancho La Puerta for a over a quarter of a century, working his way up to his present position. Like everyone else associated with Rancho La Puerta, his pride and passion are reflected in the orderly rows of produce, broken only by orchards of trees laden with fruit, that stretch as far as the eye can see. It's no wonder that Deborah absolutely insists that a visit to Tres Estrellas is a must if one is to understand the essence of her creation and the work being done by her daughter, Sarah Livia Brightwood, to ensure the continued well-being of their guests, as well as creating an educational agricultural resource for the people of Tecate through their Fundacion La Puerta.

Deborah herself is a shining example of the ultimate benefits of the healthy lifestyle she has followed for decades, full of vigour and vitality and an inspiration to all who know her. A visit to the original one-room adobe casita, now a mini-museum on the grounds of Rancho La Puerta, leaves you overwhelmed by the vast array of citations, awards and testimonials bestowed on Deborah in acknowledgement of her years of volunteerism and philanthropic work. Signatures of every president from Kennedy through George W. Bush on President's Council on Youth Fitness citations hang next to citations for her decades-long leadership in the Inter-American Foundation; her work on behalf of the arts, particularly in San Diego, and her incredible work with the children and youth on both sides of the border. They all bear testimony to the time, energy, passion and dedication of this remarkable woman, reminding you that there is still much to be done and leaving you inspired to get out there and follow her beacon.

Add to this the fact that Deborah has served as mentor to so many successful and grateful individuals in the spa business and is revered by all who know her or of her.

Deborah was kind enough to share some of her thoughts with me during a visit to Rancho La Puerta in August 2010. At 88, she was as beautiful and passionate in spirit as ever.

Deborah on Rancho La Puerta
What makes the Ranch special?

It is the amazing beauty of RLP that entices guests to breathe deep and find inner peace. Nature and its beauty, the whole environment, is part of the RLP experience. As they open up to the beauty, they open up to each other, often forming lasting friendships. When they leave, they hug and cry – exchanging email addresses and promises to write. And so many return year after year.

From the guests' comments, it's the warmth of the place. And smaller is better – a small massage room makes the experience more personal. Most guests come to spas to de-stress and it doesn't seem to be getting any better, especially with jobs being lost to the third world and people having to work harder. So we need to create an environment that helps them do that.

What is especially near and dear to your heart?

If I had a hidden agenda, it is to help guests who want their lives to be more complete find the "art" in the art of relaxation. Over the years, we have come to focus more and more on helping guests recreate and reinvent themselves to become complete and whole persons.

Life is so much more than eating, going to movies and watching TV in your spare time. It's important for our guests to discover ways of constructive, creative leisure. That's why we include classes in astronomy, weaving, photography, interpersonal relationships, and the like. We have concerts and focus on classical music. Take a look at the last thirty weeks and you'd be astonished at the variety of classes and activities we offer.

What about the future of spas?

I would hope that the world will be a better place, because of my faith in today's young persons and their ability to make it a better place. That people will come to spas for the joy of it, much as they did in ancient Rome where gladiators took the baths with senators – not so much to de-stress.

I also believe in the 3 R's: respect, responsibility and regeneration. Respect for your body by what you put into it and how you treat it. That means taking Responsibility for yourself and not depending on others to do it for you. This leads to Regeneration of the entire body and of mind and spirit.

This is what Rancho La Puerta has had at its core from the beginning and what speaks to its guests. This is what it's all about.

Thank you, Deborah.

Sheila Cluff – The Personification of Spa

Nearly twenty years after The Golden Door opened in Escondido, dynamic, Canadian-born Sheila Cluff opened the Oaks at Ojai in Ojai, California, building on her own research into exercise and nutrition and the cardiovascular fitness programs she had developed throughout the 50's and 60's.

A talented figure skater since early childhood, Sheila turned pro at the age of seventeen, touring with ice reviews and in New York shows. However, her parents insisted that she attend university, where even Sheila was not impervious to the "freshman 15" that have plagued young men and women for generations. Her petite frame went from 95 to 145 pounds in a matter of months, even though she was studying to become a physical education teacher. Alarmed, she began to look at the connection between depression and overeating and to study the correlation between emotional and physical health, recognizing that the balance of mind, body and spirit is fundamental to good health.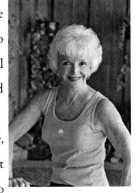

After graduating as a physical education instructor, she worked as coach in a figure skating club and taught exercise classes in which she incorporated music into her routines, for which she coined the term Cardiovascular Dance. She formed her company Fitness, Inc. as word spread and interest grew. In the meantime, she met and married her wonderful husband Don and had three children.

When Don was transferred to California to open a paper plant, Sheila was pregnant with her fourth child. Leaving behind a successful television fitness show in upstate New York, she restarted her company, Fitness Inc. and built a thriving business in Ventura County before opening The Oaks.

Throughout the 60's and into the 70's, she had continued to explore the links between nutrition, physical activity and good health, but it wasn't until she started organizing cruises to European spas that she realized that food could be both delicious and wholesome at the same time.

One of Sheila's most motivating attributes is her insistence on hiring top-notch professionals and then giving them credit where credit is due. She is the quintessential visionary who is able to galvanize and inspire others to follow her dream and one very key individual in The Oak's story is Eleanor Brown, a yoga advocate and competitive swimmer, who joined Sheila's Fitness Inc. team after moving to Ojai from Los Angeles. She had always been an advocate of fresh, healthy foods, and when her husband suffered a number of heart problems, she carefully adapted the recipes of the day to meet his physician's requirements.

When The Oaks at Ojai opened in 1977, Eleanor was made assistant manager and put in charge of the kitchen. She developed the spa's culinary offerings based on her own earlier experimentations – coupled with the increased knowledge Shelia was busy accumulating. Eleanor eventually authored a number of ever-popular cookbooks and enabled The Oaks at Ojai to set a new standard for spa cuisine that has retained its appeal to the present day. In fact, at 85, Eleanor has just completed another cookbook, *Healthy Cuisine for Singles and Doubles,* and is working on yet another!

But at The Oaks, helping Sheila's guests understand the value of healthy cuisine didn't happen overnight. Only gradually was Sheila able to convince spa patrons that a variety of fresh ingredients (with no preservatives, dyes or chemicals), prepared and served attractively, could provide the caloric values they needed to see them through a day of structured physical activity. She persevered and The Oaks at Ojai proved that spa food could be healthy and low in fat and calories without being bland and boring.

Its tag line "America's Best Spa Value" says it all, as The Oaks remains one of America's most affordable spas, reaching out to men and women of all ages interested in attaining a healthier lifestyle. Though a wonderful place to relax, the emphasis is on fitness with a wide variety of classes including cardio, yoga, dance, Pilates, mind-body, etc., plus hiking, biking, climbing and kayaking. Expert guest speakers, rounding out this preeminent destination spa's schedule of activities, lead diverse workshops held throughout the year on everything from healthy sleep to genealogy to relationship building.

Today, the award winning Oaks at Ojai continues to attract (primarily) women from around the world thanks to Sheila's goal: to help other women realize their full potential just as she has done herself. The Oaks describes its typical guest as a "fifty-year-old woman who just wants to relax and take in all the positive, nurturing elements of a healthy lifestyle" and ensures that all The

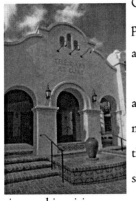

Oaks' guests receive solid tools to maintain the healthy practices they've learned through their stay at the spa – a priority and major reason for the spa's success.

Sheila's phenomenal energy and buoyant personality are every bit as evident today, as she continues to motivate and encourage those around her to realize their potential. Her generosity of spirit is legendary and she continues to lecture extensively, freely giving of her time and inspiring everyone who knows her.

At the age of 70, Sheila was approached to portray Mrs. Claus in a local skating show with 250 young children in what was to be a simple routine on ice with proceeds going to foster children in Ventura County. Sheila hadn't skated in years, but she tackled the event with the same fire and passion she brings to everything else she does, raising thousands of dollars and sparking similar charitable events in ice skating clubs across the United States. She also wound up donning her skates in earnest and four years later, in 2010, she took six firsts/golds at the Ice Skating Institute's Las Vegas national competitions.

Recently, she handed the reins as president and CEO for The Oaks and for Fitness Inc. over to her daughter, Cathy Cluff, who, after graduating with a business major from Cal Poly in San Luis Obispo in 1988, came aboard The Oaks for "one year only" and never left. For the last seven years, Cathy has served as managing director, overseeing not only day-to-day operations but also the ongoing renovations of The Oaks over the last five years. No nepotism here, as Cathy is recognized throughout the Spa industry as a leader, holding positions as president of the Destination Spa Group and vice-president of the International Spa Association Foundation's Board of Directors.

The Oaks continues to garner readers' awards from a variety of publications for everything from Most Affordable to Best Destination Spa to Best Spa Cuisine – a tribute to both the woman who hasn't hesitated to pass the baton and the younger woman ready, willing and able to pick it up and run with it.

Sharing Her Dream

Sheila says "I have supported and been interested in Wellness for years – before it was a mainstream concept – and even had set up a program with our local hospital for our guests to be tested while at The Oaks. Here in Ojai, or somewhere nearby, I envision an integrative health care clinic that would include a consortium of physicians such as a plastic surgeon, dermatologist, a Complementary and Alternative Medical Doctor and preventative medical testing related to cardiovascular disease which would work together with The Oaks and incorporate our many spa modalities as part of the overall programming.

I really see this center becoming a role model for similar centers across the country. I also see health clubs, day spas and other spas tying into their medical communities. My good friend Dr. Sharon Norling already has a similar integrative center in Westlake, MN called the Mind, Body Spirit Center and I know that it can be done."

There are a number of other individuals that have had, and continue to have, a profound impact both within the World of Spa or in the area of health and wellness: Dr. Mary Tabacchi of Cornell University; Mel and Enid Zuckerman, founders of Canyon Ranch; Susie Ellis of SpaFinder and a host of other leaders and visionaries who have dedicated themselves over the years to making Spa a household word. Each of them rates the attention and regard I have devoted to Deborah and Sheila and I salute them wholeheartedly.

As for Deborah and Sheila? What continues to amaze me as I see these two exceptional women in action is that each has remained true to her vision over the decades and that each continues to motivate the countless individuals with whom they come in contact. How exceptional is that?

Chapter 16 A Short History of Spas and Me

This final chapter comes from a purely personal perspective and I've included it because I want you to understand how spas have helped shape my life. There are many spa cultures I've left out – not because they are less significant but simply because they weren't part of my life experience. So, my apologies to any one particular group that might feel slighted!

Looking back, I realize that spa has been a part of my life from my earliest childhood.

Magical Waters of Japan

When I turned five, my father, an officer in the United States Army, was posted to Japan as part of the post-WWII "occupation forces." Dad had preceded us, leaving my mother to move a household and travel across the Pacific Ocean with two small daughters, ages five and three, on her own. In Seattle, we embarked on a US naval vessel affectionately known as the USS Mickey Mouse and enjoyed a tortuous two-week crossing as the result of having to skirt a Pacific typhoon. Nearly half the passengers were deathly ill, but we kids somehow managed to enjoy the violence of the seas and the roll of the decks beneath our feet.

Upon arriving safely in Japan, we gathered our luggage and boarded a train for Tokyo, arriving at the famous Imperial Hotel late at night. For a small child, it was all a bit overwhelming: a completely different language and culture, exotic smells and sounds, the long voyage coupled with a long train ride and the late hour. I remember feeling cold and cantankerous, to say the least, and Mother quickly agreed when the maid that had been assigned to us at the hotel suggested a bath to relax and prepare us for a good night's sleep.

That bath set the stage for a lifelong appreciation of the healing powers of water. In our room, we were given a *yukata* (cotton kimono) to wear and escorted to the hotel's communal bathhouse or *sento*. Next, we were led to a separate women's area where we sat on low stools and washed and rinsed ourselves from stem to stern. We proceeded to the baths proper and immersed ourselves in what I thought was hot water in the first tub, but that turned out to be merely the "warmer-upper." Then, upon stepping into the second bath, what followed was a miraculous and transcendent experience, thanks to the hottest water I have ever had the pleasure of bathing in, leaving us all limp and refreshed. To this day, it remains one of my most vivid memories of those early years in Japan.

It was a typical and strict protocol for bathing that remains in use even today. Before entering the baths at a *sento* or *onsen*, both men and women must first cleanse themselves with water (some offer soap), using a small towel or washcloth while sitting on a low stool. Once in the baths, the towel may not be put in or wrung out in the water. Some of the modern *onsen* feature mixed sex bathing and bathing suits are worn, but, in general, bathing is done with the same sex in the nude. While in the baths, one enjoys "naked communion" with the other bathers and a sense of community – a social phenomenon sometimes known as "skinship."

Historical Tidbits

Sento

The use of baths in Japan reaches far back into the Naro period (710-784), when they were introduced from China, and were located in temples and used for religious purposes. During the Kamakura period (1185-1333), they evolved into "hot water shops" for the general public that were also visited by sick people and thus began many of the rituals that are still in use today.

Up until the Edo period (1603-1868), women and men bathed together. However, towards the end of the Edo period, morals had become such a concern that prohibiting mixed-sex bathing was attempted several different times by the Tokugawa shogunate. They tried again after Commodore Perry's visits in 1853 and 1854, prompted by his rather vocal displeasure at the lack of morals, but to no avail. It wasn't until the Meiji period (1867-1912) in 1890, that a law was passed prohibiting mixed sex nude bathing (except for children under the age of 8 who could bathe with a parent of the opposite sex) that is still in effect to this day.

It was during the Meiji period that baths evolved into the *sento*, the communal bathhouse using heated tap water that we know today. But it was after Japan had been leveled in World War II that communal bathing and the *sento* enjoyed a real resurgence. So many homes had been destroyed during the war that public bathhouses were the only option for bathing available, with the number of *sentos* peaking in 1970.

Onsen

As part of the Pacific Ocean's "Ring of Fire," Japan is one of the most active volcanic regions in the world and home to over 2,000 mineral hot springs or *onsen*. The legal definition of an *onsen* includes that its water must contain at least one of 19 designated chemical elements, including radon and metabolic acid, and be 25°C or warmer before being reheated.[32] *Onsen* are characterized by their chemical content (iron *onsen*, sulphur *onsen*, sodium chloride *onsen*, etc.), each having a specific health benefit that is believed by the Japanese to alleviate or cure a wide variety of ailments.

While *sentos* offered the urban public the opportunity to mingle and socialize, it was the *onsen* that gave rise to the "spa vacation" as individuals and families traveled to far flung and often isolated areas to experience the health-giving geothermically heated mineral springs.

Ryokan

It is typically around *onsen* that *ryokan* flourish. These beloved traditional Japanese inns feature tatami floors, futons for sleeping and common bathing areas called *ofuro*. They are a vital part of Japan's traditional bathing culture, complementing the *onsen* by providing guests with a tranquil and structured atmosphere, as well as traditional seasonal and regional fare known as *kaiseki* — the Japanese version of spa cuisine. They can still be found in rural Japan and to a limited (and expensive!) extent in some urban settings.

Restorative Mineral Springs

When I was in my early twenties, I made a commitment to taking care of my skin, reasoning that it's the only skin I was bound to have in my lifetime and I might as well — or else wind up lined and wrinkled by the age of forty like my mother who was a sun worshipper and devoteé of good ol' soap and water.

Without understanding the underlying reasons, I embraced a daily regimen that proved to be worthwhile and that has kept my skin relatively healthy and unlined.

I hadn't even heard the concept of esthetics or the words health spa back then.

Perhaps that isn't completely accurate, because in the mid 60's my husband and I lived and worked at The Greenbrier in West Virginia — one of America's great original mineral spa hotels. Except that back then, the Greenbrier was known for its Diagnostic Clinic and the golf great, Sam Snead, rather than for its restorative water treatments. The outdoor pool was a place to relax and swim, while the indoor pool looked a bit neglected and was used rather infrequently, even on rainy summer days. I spent one entire winter as a life guard there and of the average 8-10 guests who signed in a day, the most exciting moment came when I stood face to face with Oscar Mayer of wiener and cold cuts fame!

The Greenbrier Mineral Bath Department, as it was officially known, was limited to water therapies drawing on the famous sulphur spring water for which The Greenbrier's home town of White Sulphur Springs was named. The predominantly water-based therapies included a variety of sulphur baths, scotch hose, Swiss shower and massage, but was a far cry from today's sophisticated, contemporary five-star Greenbrier Spa. After my first treatment with a scotch hose, I decided that perhaps I'd stick to swimming instead.

We used to travel to nearby Sweet Chalybeate Springs, formerly "Red" springs and famous (self-proclaimed) for having one of the highest iron contents of any springs in the world. We would pack a picnic lunch and spend an afternoon there on our days off. Though the surrounding concrete apron was old and crumbling in some places, the waters were fresh and warm at 79 degrees Fahrenheit with a whopping 800 gallons flow-through per minute. In the back of the property was a run-down building, an old hotel, whose ghostly presence recalled the prosperous heyday of the region's hot springs spas in the late 19th and early 20th century. Interestingly, there were never more than a handful of people enjoying the peaceful atmosphere and remote location.

It was Sweet Chalybeate's warm pools, surrounded by lush green grass so remarkably soft and velvety beneath our toes, that were so magical and that lured us back time and again during the two years that we called White Sulphur Springs, West Virginia home.

Historical Tidbits

The Indians of North America, who believed in the healing powers of the heat and mineral waters, considered mineral hot springs sacred places. Every major hot springs in the U.S. has some record of use by the Indians or native population, some for over 10,000 years. These springs were also known as neutral ground to which warriors could travel and rest unmolested by other tribes. There they would recuperate from battle.[33]

The Virginia Springs region of the eastern United States, with its fifteen different springs of varying chemical properties, was eventually settled by the white man. Settlers and travelers through that part of America, like the indigenous

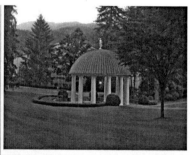

peoples before them, discovered the curative powers of these often-stinky waters and thus began the region's rich history of spas. Homesteaders understood that people would actually pay to stay and bathe in or drink the waters and, slowly, inns became hotels with the springs attracting guests from far and wide. Competition amongst the hotels gave rise to a wide variety of activities associated with modern-day resorts, so that "taking the waters" became only one facet of their offerings as they became meccas for the well-heeled socially inclined.

As time passed, The Greenbrier distinguished itself not only for its sulphur waters, but as a gathering place for some of the South's most famous southern belles, both pre and post Civil War, of whom it was said, "The Lord made the White Sulphur Springs and then the Southern girl, and rested satisfied with his work." Gentlemen were drawn to them like bees to honey and balls and cotillions were held in the Old White's splendid ballroom that caused society reporters to wax poetic.[34]

Dr. John J. Moorman, for many years the resident physician at The Greenbrier Hotel, studied the properties and attempted to define the proper usage of the White Sulphur Springs' waters. In 1854, he observed that "they are a useful remedy for Dyspepsia, Gastralgia, Water Brash, Diseases of the Liver and Spleen, Jaundice, Chronic Irritation of the Bowels, Costiveness, Piles, Diseases of the Urinary Organs, Amenorrhoea, Dysmenorrhoea and Leucorrhcea, Chronic Inflammation of the Brain, Nervous Diseases, Chronic

Diseases of the Chest, Bronchitis, Diseases of the Skin, Rheumatism and Gout, Scrofula Dropsies and Mercurial Diseases."

He went on to say, however, that "Mineral waters are not a panacea; they act like all other medicines by producing certain effects upon the animal economy, and upon principles capable of being clearly defined. It follows, that there are various diseases and states of the system to which they are not only not adapted, but in which they would be eminently injurious."[35]

Today, The Greenbrier remains a charming property, reflecting the past in style, yet very much a vibrant part of the present: a majestic white-pillared hotel on 6,500 acres in the Alleghany Mountains with 635 rooms, three championship golf courses, the magnificent 40,000 square foot Greenbrier Spa and an executive wellness clinic called The Greenbrier Center for Healthy Living.

It is also noteworthy that the nearby resort hotel, The Homestead, in Hot Springs, Virginia shares a rich history and tradition similar to that of The Greenbrier. It is home to The Jefferson Pools; is listed on America's National Register of Historic Places; is a Virginia Historic Landmark and is considered the oldest spa structure in America. Both of these two beautiful resort properties have found ways to continuously reinvent themselves over the past two centuries, reflecting the tastes and values of an ever evolving and changing population. The beauty is that they have remained at heart true to the traditions of health and southern hospitality that have defined them since they welcomed their first guests so long ago.

Kur for Health

In my late 20's, much like my mother had done so many years before, I embarked on an adventure that was to last fifteen years. We relocated our family – that now included three children under the age of six – to Germany, where my husband had decided to attempt to integrate North American business practices with the more traditional European version of hotels and hospitality.

Settling into a new culture with a young family required patience, tolerance and a willingness to adapt on my part, and adapt I did, making friends in a variety of different areas: our neighbourhood, an international women's group comprised of English, German and American women and our tennis club in those early years. Later in Bonn, Germany's capital, we became proprietors of a lovely hotel and restaurant and an integral part of the city's international scene with friends from around the world.

What fascinated me from the beginning was the German approach to health and wellness. To my surprise, the traditional medical community openly embraced many homeopathic treatments and my family physician regularly prescribed Echinacea to build up my immune system, Kneipp treatments (alternating cold and hot water) for circulatory problems, dietary restrictions for stomach maladies and even acupuncture, in addition to prescription drugs and remedies more familiar to us in North America.

Esthetics was a routine part of most women's beauty regimens, and medical pedicures for men and women (medizinische Fusspflege) could be found in every neighbourhood. Since massages were a health benefit and covered by medical insurance, massage was also a routine practice for many people. None of these practices were considered luxurious or frivolous, rather something one did in order to remain balanced and healthy. And if you got sick anyway, there was always the *Kur.*

Back in the 70's and 80's, under Germany's medical system, everyone was entitled to an all-expenses paid, two-week *Kur* in a medically supervised environment where one could do everything from undergoing a complete detox to losing weight to breathing salt air for respiratory ailments. Taking a *Kur* was exactly that: a medicinal cure for a particular medical condition or simply to improve one's immediate physical health. Relaxation was not the intent, and stress-relief was an unheard of concept. Nevertheless, friends and family would come home feeling refreshed and healthy and looking great.

There are still over 300 *Medizinische Baeder* (medical bath spas) located in every region or province in Germany. In general, when you see *Bad* in front of a town's name, it denotes a medical bath spa or town founded around some sort of springs. These *Baeder* are still highly regulated and closely monitored.

Look for the term *Luftkurort* for a climatic *Kur* that is found in the mountains, as well as at the seashore. These climatic *kurs* treat respiratory problems and allergies and are very popular, particularly for children.

The water-based (balnealogical) *Kurs* claim to treat diseases of the cardiovascular, metabolic and gastrointestinal systems; gyneacological diseases; neurological diseases; oncological diseases; psychological diseases; rheumatological diseases and diseases of the skin and urinary tract. Different *Kur* locales generally concentrate on one or a few of these different ailments with specialized clinics working together to provide the curative treatments. Inns and restaurants are part of this health network since individuals most often attend the clinics and baths on an out-patient basis rather than in a hospital setting.

It was in Germany that my eyes and mind opened by the Germans' appreciation for the health benefits provided by the healing powers of water and touch. Their respect and mainstream use of modalities that North Americans consider alternative or complementary helped to further open my eyes and heart to the "new" concept of spa that I was to encounter upon returning to North America in the late 80's.

Historical Tidbits

Roman Baths

We can thank the Romans who, as early as 200 BC, established the Roman equivalent of our modern day spas wherever they went as an integral part of their daily lives. These public bathhouses or *thermae* were built according to the bathing rituals of the day that promoted a healthy body with an emphasis on cleanliness. For men, that is.

By 33 BC, there were 170 *thermae*, public and private, in Rome alone that were very popular and frequented by most Romans. By then, women either had separate facilities or were allowed to use the full establishment at a time earlier than men, generally from dawn to one p.m., although there might be mixed bathing in the large pools.

A typical bath consisted of first preparing the body for the bath through exercise and/or an application of oils in the *unctuarium* and proceeding to the *tepidarium,* or warm room, where one warmed up and chatted with friends while scraping one's skin with a curved metal tool or *strigil.* From there it was off to the caldarium for a hot bath followed by a plunge in the cold waters of the *frigidarium.*

Refreshed, one might afterwards enjoy a massage, relax, read a book or enjoy light refreshments.

What is most important to realize is that baths had become places where business was conducted and information exchanged in a relaxed and safe environment. They were also viewed as locations for socializing and for relaxation, and even incorporated amenities such as restaurants, barber shops,

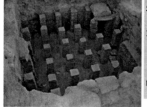

shops, masseurs and exercise areas and continued to flourish well into the 4th century AD.

Most of Europe's spas or baths were created by the Romans wherever Roman forces established a presence. In fact, Bath in England was originally known as Aquae Sulis, Baden-Baden as Aquae Aureliae and Aix-les-Bains in France as Aquae Allobrogum. This Roman legacy of famous baths has continued to draw followers unabated to the present.

Turkish Baths or Hammams

In the region of Anatolia in Turkey, the rich bathing culture of the Romans and those of Byzantium merged, combining the Roman's respect for water and the concern for cleanliness of the Moslem cultures, and developing into the hammam of today. Whether rich or poor, young or old, people of every walk of life celebrated the important milestones in their lives, from birth to death, in the hammam.

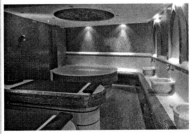

Traditional hammams can still be found not only in Turkey but also in Egypt, Morocco and other Moslem countries and were most often constructed in earliest times adjacent to mosques due to the Muslim requirement of washing face, hands and feet before praying five times a day.

It wasn't until the 18th century that the Turkish bath was introduced into Western Europe where a few have survived up to today. In 1863, Dr. Charles Shepard opened the first Turkish bath in the United States at 63 Columbia Street, Brooklyn Heights, Brooklyn[36].

In a modern Turkish bath, you enter into the *sıcaklık*, where you either sit or lie on a raised platform in the middle of the room in order to perspire freely. You then move to one of the bathing alcoves where you either wash yourself or are scrubbed, washed and massaged by an attendant. The body is first scrubbed with a coarse mitt and then lathered with a finer mitt, before being rinsed.

Bathing and resting in the warm, humid air may take from one to one and a half hours before you finally retire to the cooling-room or *soğukluk* for a period of relaxation.

Hammams, often modified to suit North American tastes, have now found their way into our North American spa culture and are here to stay.

The Social Relevance of Spa

Throughout these last few pages, have you noticed a common thread that binds all the world's great bathing traditions? From pre-recorded history to this day, they have contributed to the emotional, spiritual and physical health of their guests — not unlike the promises found in the brochures of most modern spas.

Whether a Japanese *sento*, a Roman bath, a 19th century Virginian spa, a German *Bad* or a Turkish hammam, public bathing and taking the waters has provided a means for both social interaction and relaxation. There has always been a need for safe havens where men and women can enjoy rituals associated with the restorative powers of water in the company of the same sex. It is the compelling nature of "skinship" especially in a communal setting that allows people to draw closer and genuinely relate to one another in a more profound way, enabling them to forget the cares and stresses of everyday life and find inner balance.

The communality of the spa experience is something that destination spas have always understood. Thankfully, day and resort spas are increasingly following suit. Pedicure parties, Nordic spas, the increasing popularity of hammams or even couples rooms are all geared to our desire to be able to share time together with others in a safe and nurturing environment — not so different really from the spas of yesteryear, is it?

The Last Word

Well, here we are at the end of the road and I thank you for accompanying me on this journey.

By now, you should feel confident in finding, selecting and getting the most out of your spa of choice. It's been a great deal of information, no doubt, but putting your wellbeing in someone else's hands requires a lot of trust and at least a little knowledge, so I've included as much as possible about the basics to help you on *your* spa journey. Think of all that you have learned as building blocks and a foundation for your enjoyment of everything that spas have to offer.

The more you visit spas of every type, try new treatments and deepen your understanding of what spas can do for you – mentally, spiritually and physically – the more you will find that your life has been enriched and uplifted. And it will become clear that the magic of spa is not elusive or out of reach, but can be enjoyed by all of us.

Now it's your turn to step out on your own path and discover the joys of spa for yourself.

Here's to your health!

Resource Guide

The following resources were accessed in November 2011 and represent reputable websites for up-to-date information that are not likely to become defunct. They are for your reference only and the information, recommendations and advice contained in them are not endorsed by the author or the publisher, who specifically disclaim any responsibility or liability directly or indirectly arising from their use or application. Please consult a health care professional for your particular condition or before beginning any course of treatment.

Associations

www.experienceispa.com	International Spa and Fitness Association
www.leadingspasofcanada.com	Leading Spas of Canada
www.greenspanetwork.org	Green Spa Network
www.destinationspagroup.com	Destination Spa Group
www.globalspasummit.org	Global Spa Summit

Spa Booking and Travel Blogs

www.spafinder.com	Online Booking, Guide, Club Spa
www.spasofamerica.com	Online Booking, Travel and Lifestyle blogs
www.traveltowellness.com	Spa Specials, deals, info
www.discoverspas.com	With Julie Register – Reviews, Guide
www.wayspa.com	Spa Gift Certificates (Canada)
www.sparahrah.com	Spa Travel deals

Spa Blogs

www.spas.about.com	Spas About with Anitra Brown – general info and tips
www.spaparazzi.com	Spa and Healthy Lifestyle
blog.spafinder.com	Susie Ellis' tips, spa news and trends
www.thespabuzz.com	Spa Lifestyle resource guide
www.spavelous.com	Spa directory/Locater (US)
www.spaweekblog.com	Directory, deals and discounts
www.spamagazine.com	Spa travel, beauty and Wellness
www.spaclique.com	Spa industry news of interest to professionals and consumers

Quality Assurance

www.bbb.com	Better Business Bureau
www.leadingspasofcanada.com	Quality Assurance program
www.spaquality.org	Non-industry certification

Massage

www.ncbtmb.org	National Certification Board for Therapeutic Massage and Bodywork
www.amtamassage.org	American Massage Therapy Association
www.nhpcanada.org	Association of Massage Therapists and Wholistic Practitioners
www.massage.ca	List of provincial and national Canadian Massage Therapy Associations
www.cmtbc.bc.ca	College of Massage Therapists of British Columbia
	List of medical conditions not suited for massage
www.massagemag.com	Massage Magazine

www.cmtbc.bc.ca/documents/contraindications to massage therapy April 2010.pdf

Medicine Hands: Massage Therapy for People with Cancer, Gayle MacDonald (Findhorn Press, 2007)

Massage for the Hospital Patient and Medically Frail Client, Gayle MacDonald (Lippincott Williams & Wilkins, 2005)

Hydrotherapy

www.cancer.org/Treatment/TreatmentsandSideEffects/ComplementaryandAlternativeMedicine/ManualHealingandPhysicalTouch/hydrotherapy	Info on uses and efficacy of hydrotherapy
www.spaevidence.com/spaevidence/hydrotherapy	see Spotlight for overview
http://medical-dictionary.thefreedictionary.com/hydrotherapy	Overview of hydrotherapy
www.healthline.com/galecontent/hydrotherapy	Good overview of hydrotherapy, including additional resources

The Dirt on Clean; An Unsanitized History, Katherine Aschenburg, (Alfred A. Knopf Canada, 2007)

General Health, Lifestyle and Wellness

www.mayoclinic.com	Mayo Clinic Health newsletter
www.healthywomen.org	Healthy Women newsletter and guide
www.nia.nih.gov	National Institute on Aging
www.naturalstandard.com	Integrative Medicine Newsletter
www.bravewell.org	Integrative Medicine Newsletter
www.spaevidence.com	Evidence-based research on spa modalities
www.webmd.com	General information on health and beauty issues
www.lohas.com	Lifestyles of Health and Sustainability home page
www.healinglifestyles.com	Formerly Healing Lifestyles and Spas Magazine
www.realage.com	Medical and lifestyle issues discussed by Dr. Mehmut Oz and Dr. Michael Roizen
www.DrWeil.com	Healthy aging, lifestyle and nutritional info
www.globalspasummit.org/images/stories/pdf/gss_sri_spasan	Global Spa Summit research on Spas and Wellness

dwellnessreport_rev_82010.pdf

Skin

www.rosacea-support.org	Rosacea Support Group
www.rosacea.org/patients/materials/coping/index.php	General Rosacea information on "Coping with Rosacea"
www.dove.com	Dove Skin Care
www.skincancer.org	Products, tips and info
	Sun related skin cancer information
www.webmd.com/healthy-beauty	Skin and Beauty Newsletter
www.brownskin.net/skHealth.html	Dr. Susan Taylor's Brownskin.net
www.acneguide.ca/basics/acne/what_causes_acne.html	Teen skin and acne
http://greenbeautyteam.com	Healthy and Alternative beauty tips
http://skintypesolutions.com	Dr. Leslie Baumann, MD

www.themainmeal.com.au/NR/rdonlyres/4705DAF2-6FB6-4C66-AE48-3735FB469E8A/0/Teenageacnedietbooklet_868k.pdf

Simple Skin Beauty: Every Woman's Guide to a Lifetime of Healthy, Gorgeous Skin, Dr. Ellen Marmur and Gina Way, (Atria Books, September 2009)

Sun Safety

www.fda.gov/ForConsumers/ConsumerUpdates/ucm186687.htm	Tanning facts on sunbeds, UVA, UVB and skin cancer
www.skincancer.org	Sun damage facts for all skin types/sun protection
www.SunTips.ca/index.html	B.C. Cancer Agency sun facts

www.aad.org/media-resources/stats-and-facts/prevention-and-care/sunscreens

Medical Esthetics

www.surgery.org	The American Society for Aesthetic Plastic Surgery
www.aaamed.org	The American Academy of Aesthetic Medicine
www.caam.ca	The Canadian Association of Aesthetic Medicine Physician Locator
www.yourplasticsurgeryguide.com	Consumer Guide to Plastic Surgery
www.faceinstitute.ca/index.html	The Face Institute
www.skincarephysicians.com/agingskinnet/questions_before_procedure.html	For tips on how to prepare for a cosmetic procedure
www.yourplasticsurgeryguide.com/injectables-and-fillers	For information about injectables and fillers
www.botoxcosmetic.com	Botox and Medical Providers info in your area
www.botoxcosmetic.ca	
www.plasticsurgeonslocator.com	For Board Certified Plastic Surgeons in U.S. states

www.dysport.com	Info about Dysport
www.newbeauty.com	New Beauty Magazine info on medical aesthetics, anti-aging, skin care and more

Cosmetics Ingredients

www.ewg.org/skindeep	Environmental Working Group's Skin Deep Cosmetics Database
www.cosmeticsinfo.org	Personal Care Products Council of the cosmetic, toiletry and fragrance industry
www.cosmeticscop.com/cosmetic-ingredient-dictionary	Cosmetic's Cop (Paula Begoun) ingredients dictionary
www.fda.gov/Cosmetics/ProductandIngredientSafety/SelectedCosmeticIngredients/ucm128042.htm	Parabens
www.beautypedia.com	Paula Begoun's cosmetic product information
www.healinglifestyles.com/index.php/SkinCareListings	Healing Lifestyles and Spas Magazine skin care guide

Aromatherapy

www.aromaweb.com	Guide to essential oils

Aromatherapy: An A-Z: The Most Comprehensive Guide to Aromatherapy Ever Published, Patricia Davis, (Random House UK, 2005)

The Directory of Essential Oils, Wanda Sellar, (Random House UK, 2005)

Fitness

2010_Global_Report_IHRSA.pdf	International Health, Racquet and Sportsclub Association accessed at www.globalspasummit.com
www.iayt.org	International Association of Yoga Therapists
www.incorporatingmovement.com	Pilates for Buff Bones®, Rebekah Rotstein
www.ideafit.com	IDEA Health and Fitness Association home page to find a fitness pro in your area

Body-for-LIFE for Women: A Woman's Plan for Physical and Mental Transformation, Dr. Pamela Peeke M.D. M.P.H. F.A.C.P., (Rodale Books, 2009)

Spa Nutrition

www.hc-sc.gc.ca/dhp-mps/prodnatur/about-apropos/index-eng.php	Natural Health Products Information (Health Canada)
www.stopobesityalliance.org/wp-content/themes/stopobesityalliance/pdfs/FastFacts_ObesityTrends5-2010.pdf	S.T.O.P. Obesity Alliance Fact sheet with U.S. obesity stats
www.hsph.harvard.edu/nutritionsource	The Nutrition Source newsletter published by the Harvard School of Public Health
www.fda.gov/Food/DietarySupplements/Con	Tips for the Savvy Supplement User

sumerInformation/ucm110567.htm

http://ods.od.nih.gov   Office of Dietary Supplements (NIH)

www.usp.org/aboutUSP   United States Pharmacopeial Convention international standards for food, drugs and medicine

Chef by Step – The World's Easiest Cookbook, Laurie Erickson, (Chef Laurie Publishing Co., 2010)

Cooking with the Seasons at Rancho La Puerta: Recipes from the World-Famous Spa, Deborah Szekely, Deborah Schneider and Robert Holmes (Oct 1, 2008)

The Ultimate Recipe for Fitness: Spa Cuisine from the Oaks at Ojai & the Palms at Palm Springs, Sheila Cluff, Eleanor Brown, (Fitness Pubns, June 2002)

Eating Between the Lines, Kimberly Lord Stewart, (St. Martin's Griffin, February 2007)

The Water Secret, Howard Murad, M.D., (John Wiley & Sons, 2010)

Canyon Ranch: Nourish: Indulgently Healthy Cuisine, Scott Uehlein and Canyon Ranch (Studio, Apr 16, 2009)

Encyclopedia of Nutritional Supplements, Michael Murray, ND, (Prima Publishing, 1996)

Glossaries

www.spamagazine.com/spa-glossary	List of spa terms and therapies
www.ncbtmb.org/consumers_glossary.php	Listing of massage therapies and modalities
http://experienceispa.com/spa-goers/spa-101/glossary	Listing of spa therapies and modalities
www.traveltowellness.com/spawellnessglossary	Listing of spa therapies and modalities

Magazines

http://www.spamagazine.com	6 issues per year
http://www.spalifemagazine.com	4 issues per year
http://www.spiritualityhealth.com	6 issues per year
http://www.organicspamagazine.com	7 issues per year
http://www.experiencelifemag.com	10 issues per year
http://www.shape.com	12 issues per year
http://www.self.com	12 issues per year
http://www.prevention.com	12 issues per year
http://www.eatingwell.com	6 issues per year
http://www.experienceispa.com	LiveSpa Magazine for consumers; 10 issues per year
http://www.besthealthmag.ca	7 issues per year

Acknowledgements

The idea for this book came as the result of a lunchtime conversation with my mentee, Ludvica Boota, from the University of Victoria School of Business who commented that she was looking for a "bedside" book that "tells me how to spa – in the spa and not at home." I was certain that there had to be dozens of books available on the subject and there are – on how to spa at home! But I could only find one book that actually touched on how to spa, published back in 2005.

So I started this journey – researching, interviewing, analyzing and writing, always with you, the reader in mind. It was to be about the processes of spa going in order to help people feel more comfortable and better informed about their spa time. But as I researched and analyzed, I realized that our industry is finally undergoing a major shift. Hence the book's underlying message of health and wellness.

Since I began, innumerable people have encouraged me and to all of them my most profound thanks. In particular, my daughter, Karin, has served as sounding board, proof reader, and "master of logic," while working as a full-time senior IT business analyst and still finding time to attend to the 5 horses, gaggle of turkeys, growing herd of 13 cashmere goats, 7 cats, 4 dogs, 2 mini-mules – and, I'm guessing a partridge in a pear tree – on her small 5 acre farm (with a great husband, I might add)!

My son, Rick, a talented graphics designer, gets all the credit for web-related issues, book layout and cover design, all done while working as an investment advisor and being a dedicated and supportive father to three active teenagers. It's truly been a family affair.

My deepest thanks to all those along the way who have shared their wisdom and knowledge: for the book's wonderful foreword by Susie Ellis, woman extraordinaire who has the fastest email response time of anyone I know and is both smart and beautiful in equal measure; my friend Ellen Coburn, for all her help proofing the chapters on massage and skin care; Jeff Kohl, for his illuminating discourse on network fitness; Lynne McNees, president of the International Spa Association, for comments and suggestions that helped round out this book; Chef Laurie Erickson for her input on spa cuisine; Maureen Rutherford, representative for Allergan, Inc., for a passionate description of the proper uses of Botox®; Dr. Mark Lupin, MD, FRCPC, who freely gave me hours of his time to talk about medical aesthetic spa treatments and the importance of medical doctors in medical spas; Dr. Wendy Smeltzer, longtime friend and colleague, for her contributions; my son-in-law Rick Carlsen for a real man's reaction to the chapter on men; my daughter, Kristy, who between work and two toddlers still took the time to listen and advise; for the warm hospitality shown to me and my husband by Rancho La Puerta and Deborah Szekely; for the phone calls and interviews with my dear friend Sheila Cluff; and most especially to my wonderfully patient husband, Rick, who nodded dutifully every time I said "Now, I've finished the book!"

Stock Photo Images are licensed through Shutterstock® or are the author's.

Endnotes

[1] http://www.coylehospitality.com/research_reports/coyle-hospitality-group-wts-international-spa-sentiment-research-report-2009/ accessed November 2011

[2] http://www6.miami.edu/touch-research/About.html accessed October 2011

[3] Mark Hyman Rapaport, Pamela Schettler, Catherine Bresee. The Journal of Alternative and Complementary Medicine. Volume 16, Number 10, 2010, pp.1-10

[4] "The Electricity of Touch: Detection and Measurement of Cardiac Energy Exchange Between People" Rollin McCraty, Ph.D., Mike Atkinson, Dana Tomasino, B.A., and William A. Tiller, Ph.D. in: Karl H. Pribram, ed. Brain and Values: Is a Biological Science of Values Possible. Mahwah, NJ: Lawrence Erlbaum Associates, Publishers, 1998: 359-379.

[5] http://www.massagetoday.com/mpacms/mt/article.php?id=10245, Kate Jordan, NCTMB accessed October 2011

[6] http://www.skincarephysicians.com/agingskinnet/basicfacts.html accessed November 2011

[7] LK Heilbronn, E Ravussin, Calorie restriction and aging: review of the literature and implications for studies in humans. Amer J Clin Nutr 78(3) 361–369 (2003)

[8] Anti-collagenase, anti-elastase and anti-oxidant activities of extracts from 21 plants, Tamsyn SA Thring and Declan Naughton, School of Life Sciences, Kingston University, London, KT1 2EE, UK and Pauline Hili, Neal's Yard Remedies, 15 Neal's Yard, London, WC2H 9DP, UK BMC Complementary and Alternative Medicine 2009, 9:27doi:10.1186/1472-6882-9-27

[9] "Resveratrol: A Real Anti-aging Product," Peter T. Pugliese, MD, Skin Inc. Magazine, December 2008 accessed Novemer 2011

[10] http://www.medicalnewstoday.com/articles/72129.php

[11] http://www.brownskin.net/skHealth.html accessed September 2011

[12] I. Smith, R., Mann, N., Braue, A., Makalainen, H. and Varigos, G. "The effect of a higher protein, low glycaemic load diet vs a conventional, high glycaemic load diet on biochemical parameters associated with acne vulgaris. A randomised, investigator-masked, controlled trial." Journal of the American Academy of Dermatology (in press).

[13] http://www.rosacea.org/patients/allaboutrosacea.php accessed October 2011

[14] http://www.skincancer.org/For-Parents/ accessed November 2011

[15] http://www.skincancer.org/skin-cancer-and-skin-of-color.html accessed November 2011

[16] http://www.SunTips.ca/index.html , BC Cancer Agency, 2008 accessed November 2011

[17] http://www.skincancer.org/understanding-uva-and-uvb.html accessed November 2011

[18] http://www.medicalnewstoday.com/articles/189656.php, "New Survey Exposes The Most Common Myths About Tanning And Sun Protection", May 24, 2010 accessed November 2011

[19] http://www.accessdata.fda.gov/cms_ia/importalert_127.html accessed November 2011

[20] ISPA 2010 US Spa Industry Study, International Spa Association, p.66

[21]http://www.fda.gov/Cosmetics/ProductandIngredientSafety/ProductInformation/ucm127068.htm

[22] http://nccam.nih.gov/health/whatiscam/ accessed September 2011

[23] http://www.ahc.umn.edu/cahcim/about/home.html accessed September 2011

[24] 2010 Complementary and Alternative Medicine Survey of Hospitals Summary of Results, Sita Ananth, MHA, Samueli Institute, September 2011

[25] http://www.bravewell.org/integrative_medicine/patient_rights/ accessed November 2011

[26] http://www.ahc.umn.edu/cahcim/about/home.html accessed November 2011

[27] http://e-patients.net/e-Patients_White_Paper.pdf accessed November 2011

[28] http://www.drpeeke.com/

[29] Global Spa Summit, Spas and the Global Wellness Market: Synergies and Opportunities, prepared by SRI International, May 2010) available at http://www.globalspasummit.org/index.php/spa-industry-resource

[30] http://www.cdc.gov/obesity/causes/economics.html

[31] ISPA 2010 US Spa Industry Study, International Spa Association, p.73

[32] http://en.wikipedia.org/wiki/Onsen

[33] Balneological Use of Geothermal Waters, pdf. John W. Lund, International Summer School on Direct Application of Geothermal Energy

[34] The Greenbrier Heritage, William Olcott, the Netherlands, 1965

[35] The Virginia Springs : comprising an account of all the principal mineral springs of Virginia, with remarks on the nature and medical applicability of each; Dr. John J. Moorman

[36] http://en.wikipedia.org/wiki/Turkish_bath accessed November 2011

CPSIA information can be obtained at www.ICGtesting.com
Printed in the USA
LVOW102208281012

304780LV00004BA/1/P